Poultry With A Mediterranean Twist

Fresh Recipes to Boost Your Poultry Game

By
Delia Bell

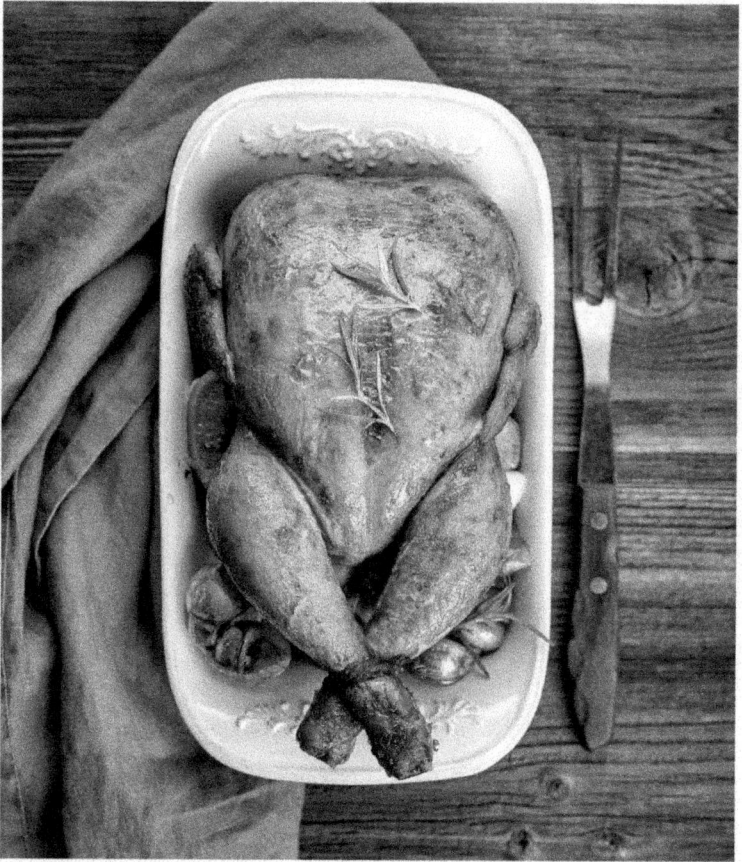

solely under their purview. There are no scenarios in which the publisher or the original author of this work can be in any fashion deemed liable for any hardship or damages that may befall them after undertaking information described herein.

Additionally, the information in the following pages is intended only for informational purposes and should thus be thought of as universal. As befitting its nature, it is presented without assurance regarding its prolonged validity or interim quality. Trademarks that are mentioned are done without written consent and can in no way be considered an endorsement from the trademark holder.

Table of Contents

INTRODUCTION

What is the Mediterranean Diet?

The Mediterranean diet is based on the diets of traditional eating habits from the 1960s of people from countries that surround the Mediterranean Sea, such as Greece, Italy, and Spain, and it encourages the consumption of fresh, seasonal, and local foods. The Mediterranean diet has become popular because individuals show low rates of heart disease, chronic disease, and obesity. The Mediterranean diet profile focuses on whole grains, good fats (fish, olive oil, nuts etc.), vegetables, fruits, fish, and very low consumption of any non-fish meat. Along with food, the Mediterranean diet emphasizes the need to spend time eating with family and physical activity. The Mediterranean diet is not a single prescribed diet, but rather a general food-based eating pattern, which is marked by local and cultural differences throughout the Mediterranean region.

The diet is generally characterized by a high intake of plant-based foods (e.g. fresh fruit and vegetables, nuts, and cereals) and olive oil, a moderate intake of fish and poultry, and low intakes of dairy products (mostly yoghurt and cheese), red and processed meats, and sweets. Wine is typically consumed in moderation and, normally, with a meal. A strong focus is placed on social and cultural aspects, such as communal mealtimes, resting after eating, and regular physical activity. Nowadays, however, the diet is no longer followed as widely as it was 30-50 years ago, as the diets of people living in these regions are becoming more 'Westernized' and higher in energy dense foods.

Benefits

The Mediterranean diet is not a weight loss, but increasing fiber intake and cutting out red meat, animal fats, and processed food may lead to weight loss. People who follow the diet may also have a lower risk of various diseases.

Heart health

In the 1950s,an American scientist, found that people living in the poorer areas of southern Italy had a lower risk of heart disease and death than those in wealthier parts of New York. Dr. Keys attributed this to diet. Since then, many studies have indicated that following a Mediterranean diet can help the body maintain healthy cholesterol levels and reduce the risk of high blood pressure and cardiovascular disease. The overall pattern of the Mediterranean diet is similar to their own dietary recommendations. A high proportion of calories on the diet come from fat, which can increase the risk of obesity. However, they also note that this fat is mainly unsaturated, which makes it a more healthful option than that from the typical American diet.

Protection from disease

The Mediterranean diet focuses on plant-based foods, and these are good sources of antioxidants.

The Mediterranean diet might offer protection from various cancers, and especially colorectal cancer. The reduction in risk may stem from the high intake of fruits, vegetables, and whole grains. By sticking to Mediterranean meals, people's levels of blood glucose and fats had decreased. During this time, there was also a lower incidence of stroke.

Diabetes
The Mediterranean diet may help prevent type 2 diabetes and improve markers of diabetes in people who already have the condition. Various other studies have concluded that following the Mediterranean diet can reduce the risk of type 2 diabetes and cardiovascular disease, which often occur together.

Food to eat
There is no single definition of the Mediterranean diet, but one group of scientists used the following as their 2015 basis of research.

Vegetables: Include 3 to 9 servings a day.

Fresh fruit: Up to 2 servings a day.

Cereals: Mostly whole grain from 1 to 13 servings a day.

Oil: Up to 8 servings of extra virgin (cold pressed) olive oil a day.

Fat — mostly unsaturated — made up 37% of the total calories. Unsaturated fat comes from plant sources, such as olives and avocado. The Mediterranean diet also provided 33 grams (g) of fiber a day. The baseline diet for this study provided around

2,200 calories a day. Typical ingredients. Here are some examples of ingredients that people often include in the Mediterranean diet.

Vegetables: Tomatoes, peppers, onions, eggplant, zucchini, cucumber, leafy green vegetables, plus others.

Fruits: Melon, apples, apricots, peaches, oranges, and lemons, and so on.

Legumes: Beans, lentils, and chickpeas.

Nuts and seeds: Almonds, walnuts, sunflower seeds, and cashews.

Unsaturated fat: Olive oil, sunflower oil, olives, and avocados.

Dairy products: Cheese and yogurt are the main dairy foods.

Cereals: These are mostly whole grain and include wheat and rice with bread accompanying many meals.

Fish: Sardines and other oily fish, as well as oysters and other shellfish. Poultry: Chicken or turkey.

Eggs: Chicken, quail, and duck eggs.

Drinks: A person can drink red wine in moderation.

The Mediterranean diet does not include strong liquor or carbonated and sweetened drinks. According to one definition, the diet limits red meat and sweets to less than 2 servings per week.

Food to avoid

Here's a list of foods you should generally limit while eating Mediterranean-style meals. Heavily processed foods. Let's be real: Many, many foods are processed to some degree. A can of beans has been processed, in the sense that the beans have been cooked before being canned. Olive oil has been processed, because olives have been turned into oil. But when we talk about limiting processed foods, this really means avoiding things like frozen meals with tons of sodium. You should also limit soda, desserts and candy. As the adage goes, if the ingredient list includes items that your great-grandparents wouldn't recognize as food, it's probably processed. If you're buying a packaged food that's as close to its whole-food form as possible — such as frozen fruit or veggies with nothing added — you're good to go.

Processed red meat

On the Mediterranean diet, you should minimize your intake of red meat, such as steak. What about processed red meat, such as hot dogs and bacon? You should avoid these foods or limit them as much as possible. A study published in BMJ found that regularly eating red meat, especially processed varieties, was associated with a higher risk of death. Butter. Here's another food that should be limited on the Mediterranean diet. Use olive oil instead, which has many heart health benefits and contains less saturated fat than butter. According to the USDA National Nutrient Database, butter has 7 grams of saturated fat per tablespoon, while olive oil has about 2 grams.

Refined grains

The Mediterranean diet is centered around whole grains, such as farro, millet, couscous and brown rice. With this eating style, you'll generally want to limit your intake of refined grains such as white pasta and white bread.

Alcohol

When you're following the Mediterranean diet, red wine should be your chosen alcoholic drink. This is because red wine offers health benefits, particularly for the heart. But it's important to limit intake of any type of alcohol to up to one drink per day for women, as well as men older than 65, and up to two drinks daily for men age 65 and younger. The amount that counts as a drink is 5 ounces of wine, 12 ounces of beer or 1.5 ounces of 80-proof liquor.

Chili Chicken Mix

Servings: 4

Cooking Time: 18 Minutes

Ingredients:

- 2 pounds chicken thighs, skinless and boneless
- 2 tablespoons olive oil
- 2 cups yellow onion, chopped
- 1 teaspoon onion powder
- 1 teaspoon smoked paprika
- 1 teaspoon chili pepper
- ½ teaspoon coriander seeds, ground
- 2 teaspoons oregano, dried
- 2 teaspoon parsley flakes
- 30 ounces canned tomatoes, chopped
- ½ cup black olives, pitted and halved

Directions:

1. Set the instant pot on Sauté mode, add the oil, heat it up, add the onion,
onion powder and the rest of the ingredients except the tomatoes, olives and the chicken, stir and sauté for 10 minutes.

2. Add the chicken, tomatoes and the olives, put the lid on and cook on High for 8 minutes.

3. Release the pressure naturally for 10 minutes, divide the mix into bowls and serve.

Nutrition Info: calories 153, fat 8, fiber 2, carbs 9, protein 12

Ginger Duck Mix

Servings: 4

Cooking Time: 1 Hour And 50 Minutes

Ingredients:

- 4 duck legs, boneless
- 4 shallots, chopped
- 2 tablespoons olive oil
- 1 tablespoon ginger, grated
- 2 tablespoons rosemary, chopped
- 1 cup chicken stock
- 1 tablespoon chives, chopped

Directions:

1. In a roasting pan, combine the duck legs with the shallots and the rest of the ingredients except the chives, toss, introduce in the oven at 250 degrees F and bake for 1 hour and 30 minutes.

2. Divide the mix between plates, sprinkle the chives on top and serve.

Nutrition Info: calories 299, fat 10.2, fiber 9.2, carbs 18.1, protein 17.3

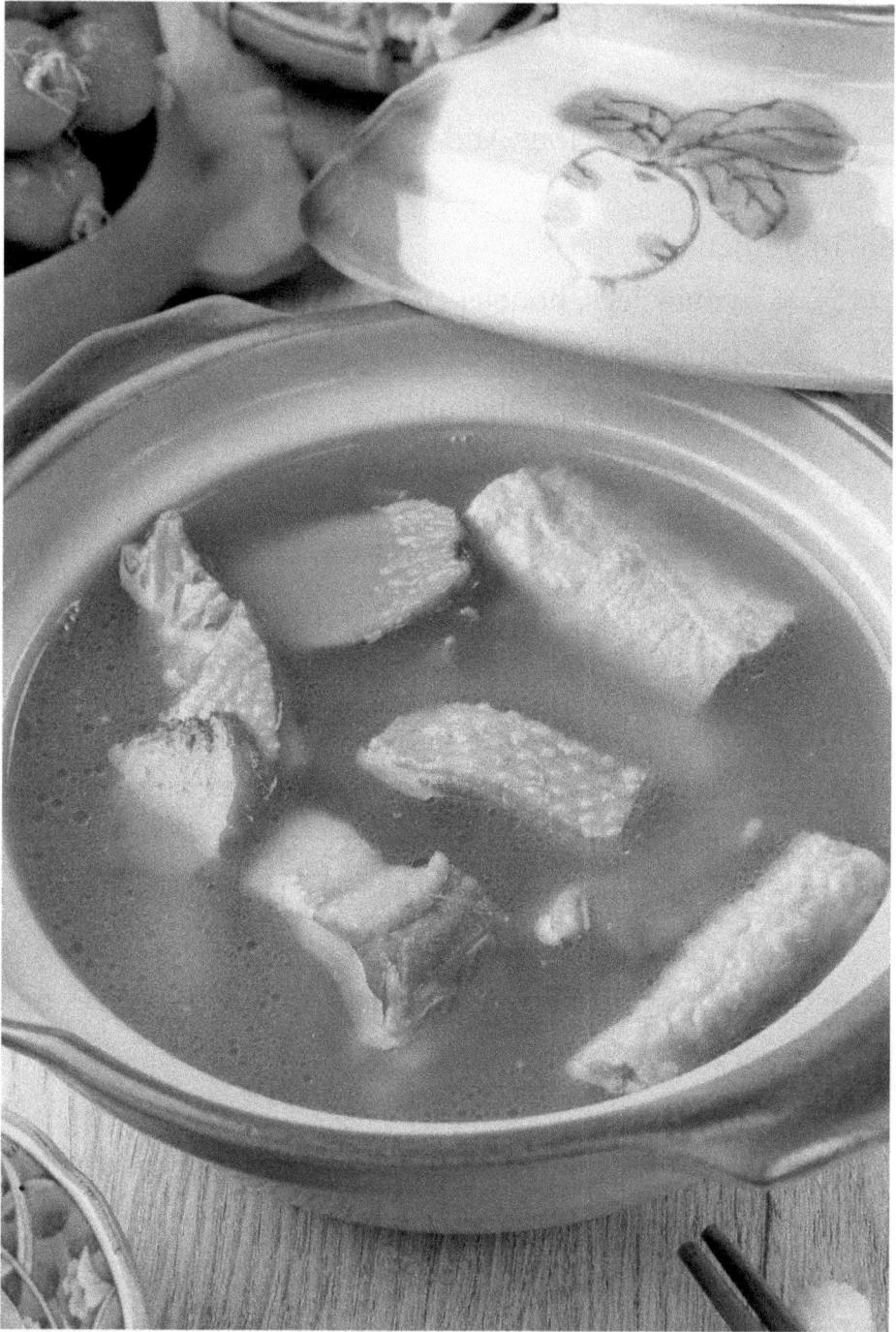

Duck And Orange Warm Salad

Servings: 4

Cooking Time: 25 Minutes

Ingredients:

- 2 tablespoons balsamic vinegar
- 2 oranges, peeled and cut into segments
- 1 teaspoon orange zest, grated
- 1 tablespoons orange juice
- 3 shallot, minced
- 2 tablespoons olive oil
- Salt and black pepper to the taste
- 2 duck breasts, boneless and skin scored
- 2 cups baby arugula
- 2 tablespoons chives, chopped

Directions:

1. Heat up a pan with the oil over medium-high heat, add the duck breasts skin side down and brown for 5 minutes.

2. Flip the duck, add the shallot, and the other ingredients except the arugula, orange and the chives, and cook for 15 minutes more.

3. Transfer the duck breasts to a cutting board, cool down, cut into strips and put in a salad bowl.

4. Add the remaining ingredients, toss and serve warm.

Nutrition Info: calories 304, fat 15.4, fiber 12.6, carbs 25.1, protein 36.4

Turmeric Baked Chicken Breast

Servings: 2

Cooking Time: 40 Minutes

Ingredients:
- 8 oz chicken breast, skinless, boneless
- 2 tablespoons capers
- 1 teaspoon olive oil
- ½ teaspoon paprika
- ½ teaspoon ground turmeric
- ½ teaspoon salt
- ½ teaspoon minced garlic

Directions:

1. Make the lengthwise cut in the chicken breast.

2. Rub the chicken with olive oil, paprika, capers, ground turmeric, salt, and minced garlic.

3. Then fill the chicken cut with capers and secure it with the toothpicks.

4. Bake the chicken breast for 40 minutes at 350F.

5. Remove the toothpicks from the chicken breast and slice it.

Nutrition Info:Per Serving:calories 156, fat 5.4, fiber 0.6, carbs 1.3, protein 24.4

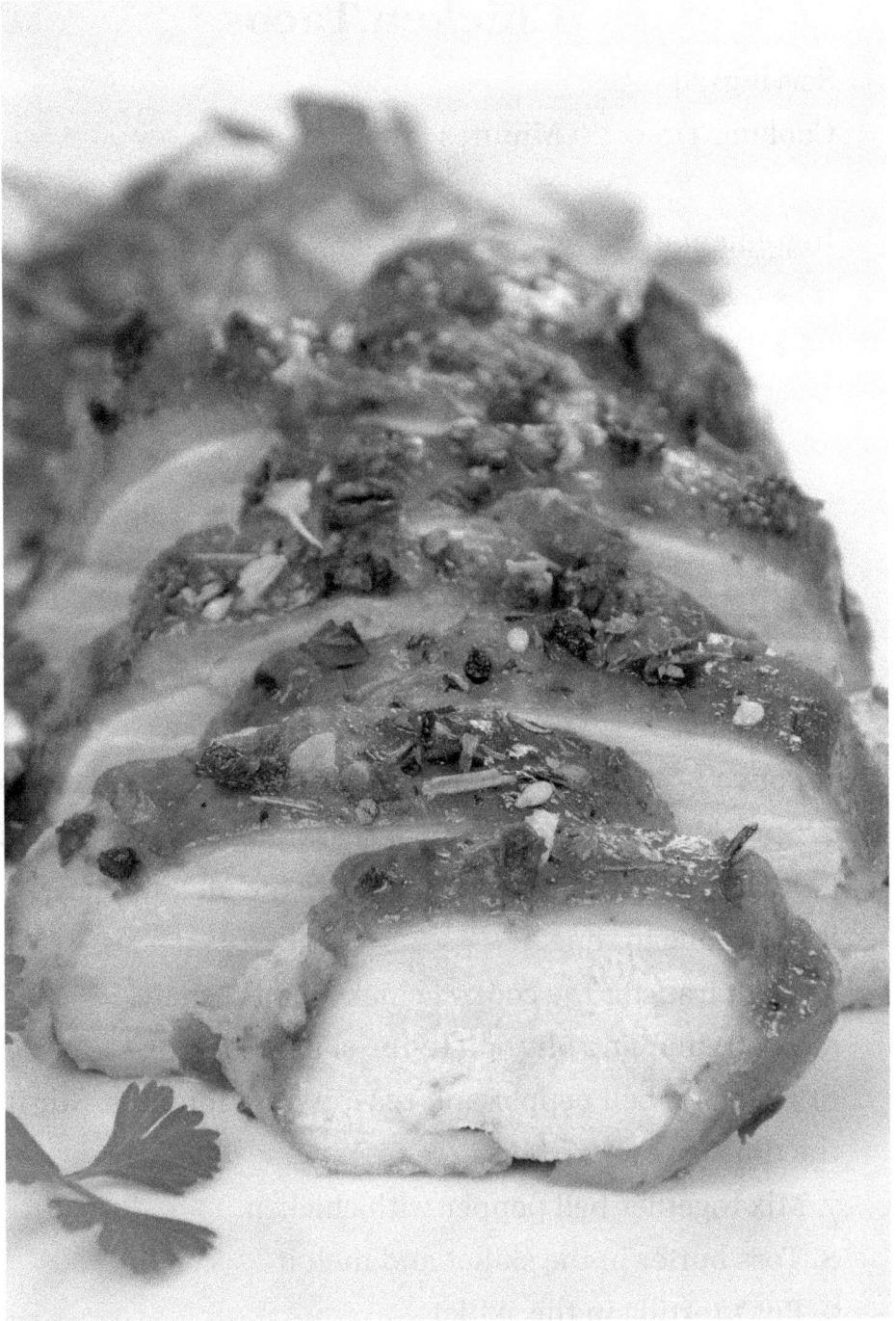

Chicken Tacos

Servings: 4

Cooking Time: 20 Minutes

Ingredients:
- 2 bread tortillas
- 1 teaspoon butter
- 2 teaspoons olive oil
- 1 teaspoon Taco seasoning
- 6 oz chicken breast, skinless, boneless, sliced
- 1/3 cup Cheddar cheese, shredded
- 1 bell pepper, cut on the wedges

Directions:

1. Pour 1 teaspoon of olive oil in the skillet and add chicken.

2. Sprinkle the meat with Taco seasoning and mix up well.

3. Roast chicken for 10 minutes over the medium heat. Stir it from time to time.

4. Then transfer the cooked chicken to the plate.

5. Add remaining olive oil in the skillet.

6. Then add bell pepper and roast it for 5 minutes. Stir it all the time.

7. Mix together bell pepper with chicken.

8. Toss butter in the skillet and melt it.

9. Put 1 tortilla in the skillet.

10. Put Cheddar cheese on the tortilla and flatten it.

11. Then add chicken-pepper mixture and cover it with the second tortilla.

12. Roast the quesadilla for 2 minutes from each side.

13. Cut the cooked meal on the halves and transfer in the serving plates.

Nutrition Info:Per Serving:calories 194, fat 8.3, fiber 0.6, carbs 16.4, protein 13.2

Chicken And Butter Sauce

Servings: 5

Cooking Time: 30 Minutes

Ingredients:

- 1-pound chicken fillet
- 1/3 cup butter, softened
- 1 tablespoon rosemary
- ½ teaspoon thyme
- 1 teaspoon salt
- ½ lemon

Directions:

1. Churn together thyme, salt, and rosemary.

2. Chop the chicken fillet roughly and mix up with churned butter mixture.

3. Place the prepared chicken in the baking dish.

4. Squeeze the lemon over the chicken.

5. Chop the squeezed lemon and add in the baking dish.

6. Cover the chicken with foil and bake it for 20 minutes at 365F.

7. Then discard the foil and bake the chicken for 10 minutes more.

Nutrition Info:Per Serving:calories 285, fat 19.1, fiber 0.5, carbs 1, protein 26.5

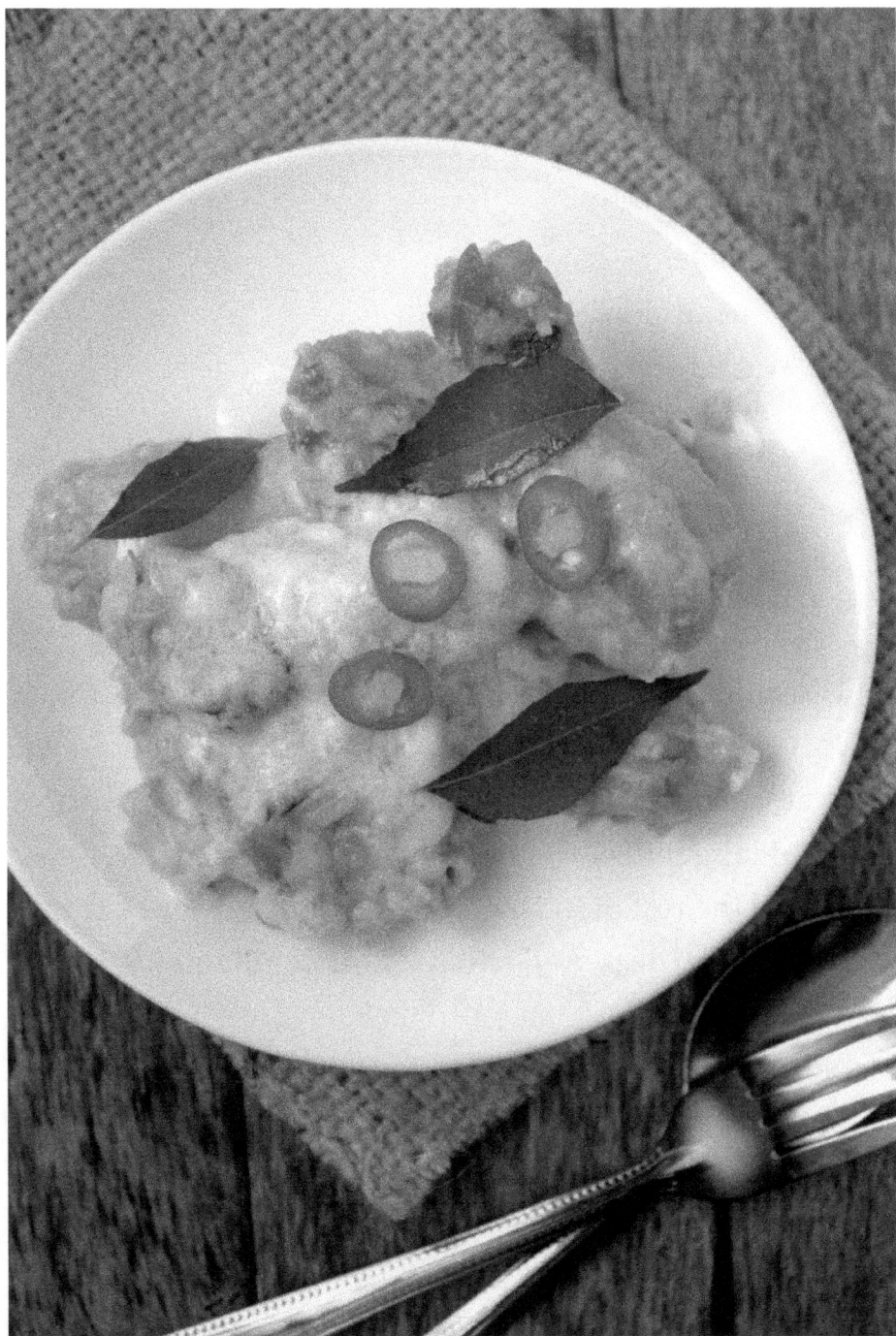

Turkey And Cranberry Sauce

Servings: 4

Cooking Time: 50 Minutes

Ingredients:

- 1 cup chicken stock
- 2 tablespoons avocado oil
- ½ cup cranberry sauce
- 1 big turkey breast, skinless, boneless and sliced
- 1 yellow onion, roughly chopped
- Salt and black pepper to the taste

Directions:

1. Heat up a pan with the avocado oil over medium-high heat, add the onion and sauté for 5 minutes.
2. Add the turkey and brown for 5 minutes more.
3. Add the rest of the ingredients, toss, introduce in the oven at 350 degrees F and cook for 40 minutes

Nutrition Info: calories 382, fat 12.6, fiber 9.6, carbs 26.6, protein 17.6

Coriander And Coconut Chicken

Servings: 4

Cooking Time: 30 Minutes

Ingredients:

- 2 pounds chicken thighs, skinless, boneless and cubed
- 2 tablespoons olive oil
- Salt and black pepper to the taste
- 3 tablespoons coconut flesh, shredded
- 1 and ½ teaspoons orange extract
- 1 tablespoon ginger, grated
- ¼ cup orange juice
- 2 tablespoons coriander, chopped
- 1 cup chicken stock
- ¼ teaspoon red pepper flakes

Directions:

1. Heat up a pan with the oil over medium-high heat, add the chicken and brown for 4 minutes on each side.
2. Add salt, pepper and the rest of the ingredients, bring to a simmer and cook over medium heat for 20 minutes.
3. Divide the mix between plates and serve hot.

Nutrition Info: calories 297, fat 14.4, fiber 9.6, carbs 22, protein 25

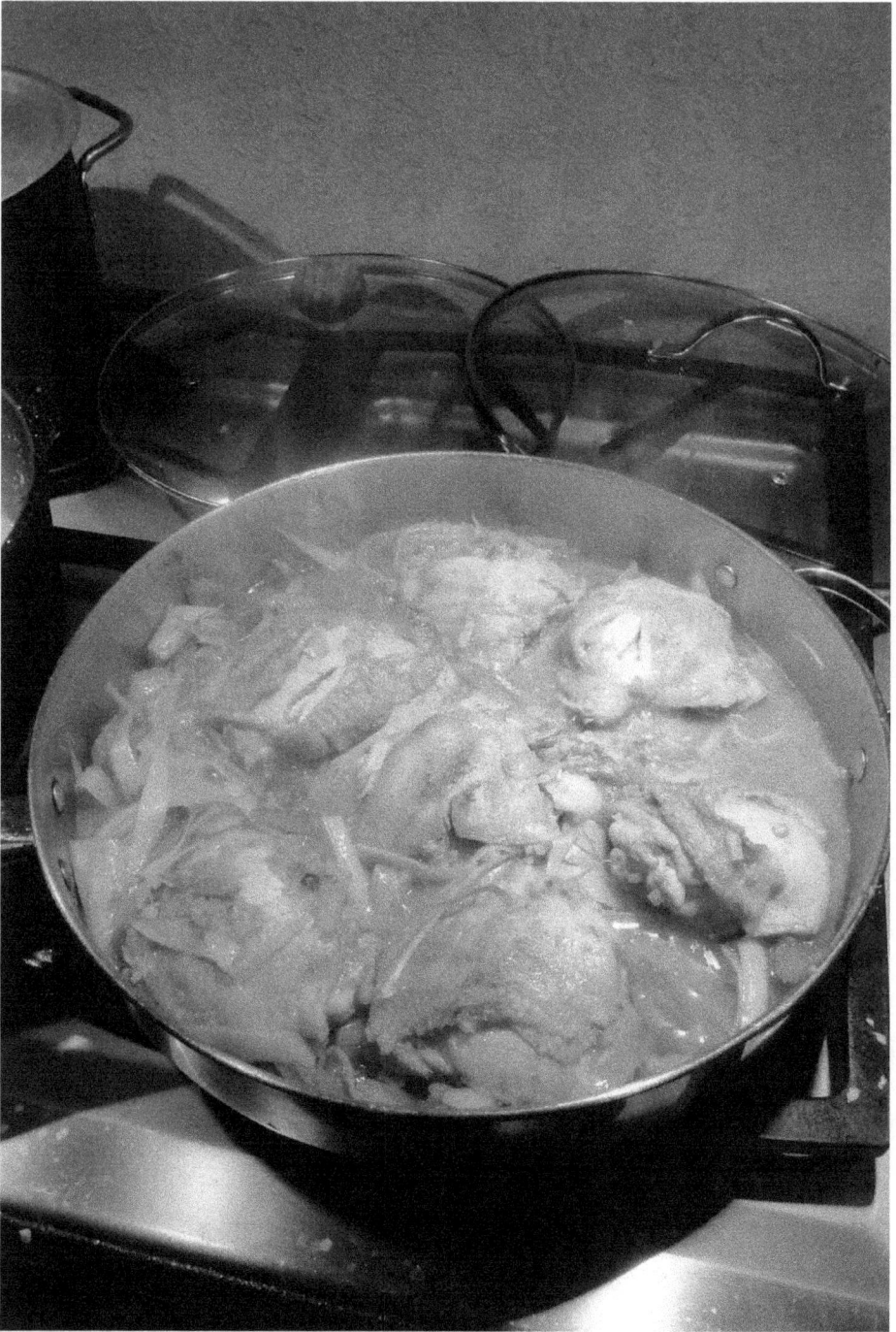

Chicken Pilaf

Servings: 4

Cooking Time: 30 Minutes

Ingredients:

- 4 tablespoons avocado oil
- 2 pounds chicken breasts, skinless, boneless and cubed
- ½ cup yellow onion, chopped
- 4 garlic cloves, minced
- 8 ounces brown rice
- 4 cups chicken stock
- ½ cup kalamata olives, pitted
- ½ cup tomatoes, cubed
- 6 ounces baby spinach
- ½ cup feta cheese, crumbled
- A pinch of salt and black pepper
- 1 tablespoon marjoram, chopped
- 1 tablespoon basil, chopped
- Juice of ½ lemon
- ¼ cup pine nuts, toasted

Directions:

1. Heat up a pot with 1 tablespoon avocado oil over medium-high heat, add the chicken, some salt and pepper, brown for 5 minutes on each side and transfer to a bowl.

2. Heat up the pot again with the rest of the avocado oil over medium heat, add the onion and garlic and sauté for 3 minutes.

3. Add the rice, the rest of the ingredients except the pine nuts, also return the chicken, toss, bring to a simmer and cook over medium heat for 20 minutes.

4. Divide the mix between plates, top each serving with some pine nuts and serve.

Nutrition Info: calories 283, fat 12.5, fiber 8.2, carbs 21.5, protein 13.4

Chicken And Black Beans

Servings: 4

Cooking Time: 20 Minutes

Ingredients:

- 12 oz chicken breast, skinless, boneless, chopped
- 1 tablespoon taco seasoning
- 1 tablespoon nut oil
- ½ teaspoon cayenne pepper
- ½ teaspoon salt
- ½ teaspoon garlic, chopped
- ½ red onion, sliced
- 1/3 cup black beans, canned, rinsed
- ½ cup Mozzarella, shredded

Directions:

1. Rub the chopped chicken breast with taco seasoning, salt, and cayenne pepper.

2. Place the chicken in the skillet, add nut oil and roast it for 10 minutes over the medium heat. Mix up the chicken pieces from time to time to avoid burning.

3. After this, transfer the chicken in the plate.

4. Add sliced onion and garlic in the skillet. Roast the vegetables for 5 minutes. Stir them constantly. Then add

black beans and stir well. Cook the ingredients for 2 minute more.

5. Add the chopped chicken and mix up well. Top the meal with Mozzarella cheese.

6. Close the lid and cook the meal for 3 minutes.

Nutrition Info:Per Serving:calories 209, fat 6.4, fiber 2.8, carbs 13.7, 22.7

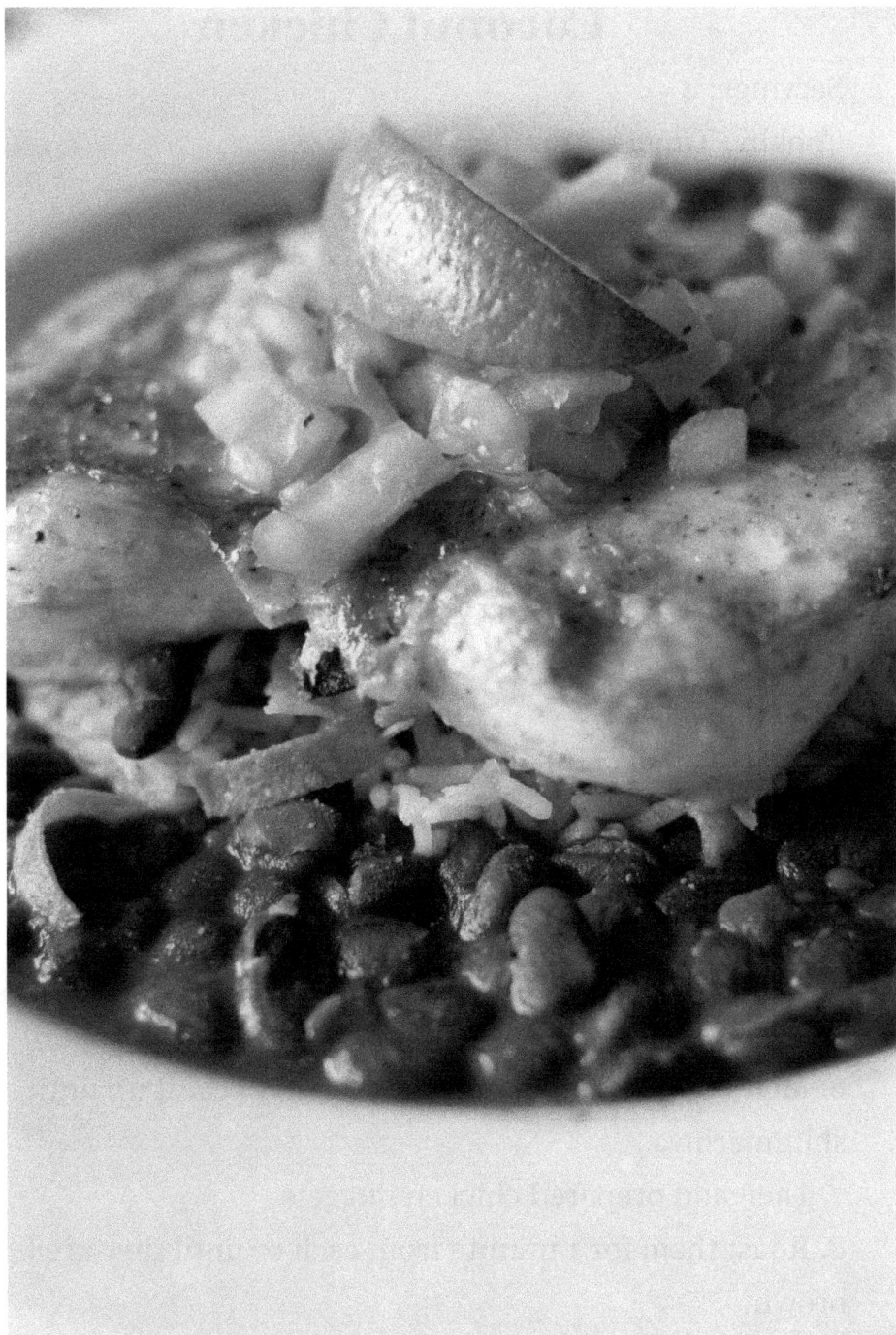

Coconut Chicken

Servings: 4

Cooking Time: 5 Minutes

Ingredients:
- 6 oz chicken fillet
- ¼ cup of sparkling water
- 1 egg
- 3 tablespoons coconut flakes
- 1 tablespoon coconut oil
- 1 teaspoon Greek Seasoning

Directions:

1. Cut the chicken fillet on small pieces (nuggets).

2. Then crack the egg in the bowl and whisk it.

3. Mix up together egg and sparkling water.

4. Add Greek seasoning and stir gently.

5. Dip the chicken nuggets in the egg mixture and then coat in the coconut flakes.

6. Melt the coconut oil in the skillet and heat it up until it is shimmering.

7. Then add prepared chicken nuggets.

8. Roast them for 1 minute from each or until they are light brown.

9. Dry the cooked chicken nuggets with the help of the paper towel and transfer in the serving plates.

Nutrition Info:Per Serving:calories 141, fat 8.9, fiber 0.3, carbs 1, protein 13.9

Ginger Chicken Drumsticks

Servings: 4

Cooking Time: 30 Minutes

Ingredients:

- 4 chicken drumsticks
- 1 apple, grated
- 1 tablespoon curry paste
- 4 tablespoons milk
- 1 teaspoon coconut oil
- 1 teaspoon chili flakes
- ½ teaspoon minced ginger

Directions:

1. Mix up together grated apple, curry paste, milk, chili flakes, and minced garlic.
2. Put coconut oil in the skillet and melt it.
3. Add apple mixture and stir well.
4. Then add chicken drumsticks and mix up well.
5. Roast the chicken for 2 minutes from each side.
6. Then preheat oven to 360F.
7. Place the skillet with chicken drumsticks in the oven and bake for 25 minutes.

Nutrition Info:Per Serving:calories 150, fat 6.4, fiber 1.4, carbs 9.7, protein 13.5

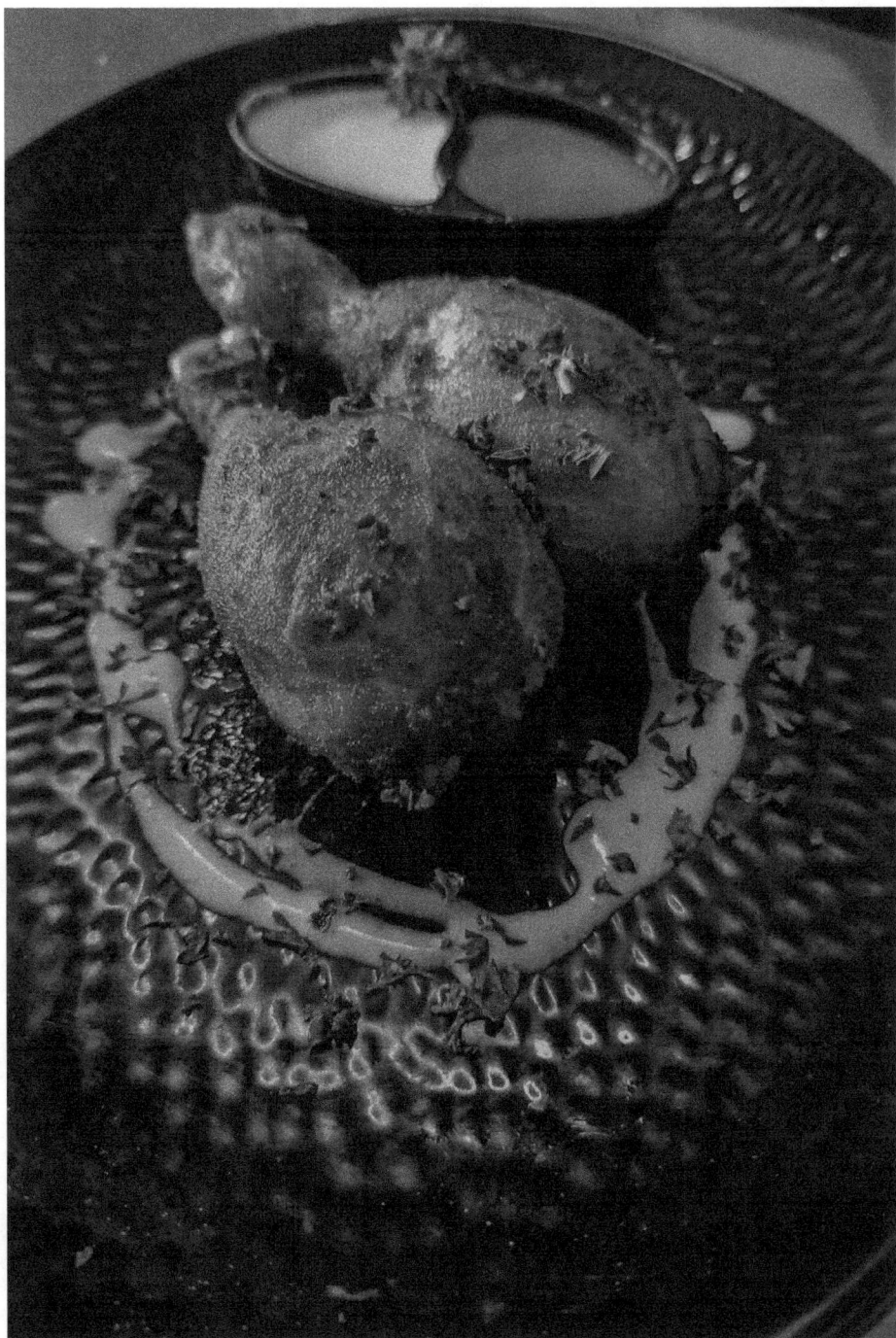

Parmesan Chicken

Servings: 3

Cooking Time: 30 Minutes

Ingredients:

- 1-pound chicken breast, skinless, boneless
- 2 oz Parmesan, grated
- 1 teaspoon dried oregano
- ½ teaspoon dried cilantro
- 1 tablespoon Panko bread crumbs
- 1 egg, beaten
- 1 teaspoon turmeric

Directions:

1. Cut the chicken breast on 3 servings.

2. Then combine together Parmesan, oregano, cilantro, bread crumbs, and turmeric.

3. Dip the chicken servings in the beaten egg carefully.

4. Then coat every chicken piece in the cheese-bread crumbs mixture.

5. Line the baking tray with the baking paper.

6. Arrange the chicken pieces in the tray.

7. Bake the chicken for 30 minutes at 365F.

Nutrition Info:Per Serving:calories 267, fat 9.5, fiber 0.5, carbs 3.2, protein 40.4

Pomegranate Chicken

Servings: 6

Cooking Time: 25 Minutes

Ingredients:
- 1-pound chicken breast, skinless, boneless
- 1 tablespoon za'atar
- ½ teaspoon salt
- 1 tablespoon pomegranate juice
- 1 tablespoon olive oil

Directions:

1. Rub the chicken breast with za'atar seasoning, salt, olive oil, and pomegranate juice.

2. Marinate the chicken or 15 minutes and transfer in the skillet.

3. Roast the chicken for 15 minutes over the medium heat.

4. Then flip the chicken on another side and cook for 10 minutes more.

5. Slice the chicken and place in the serving plates.

Nutrition Info:Per Serving:calories 107, fat 4.2, fiber 0, carbs 0.2, protein 16.1

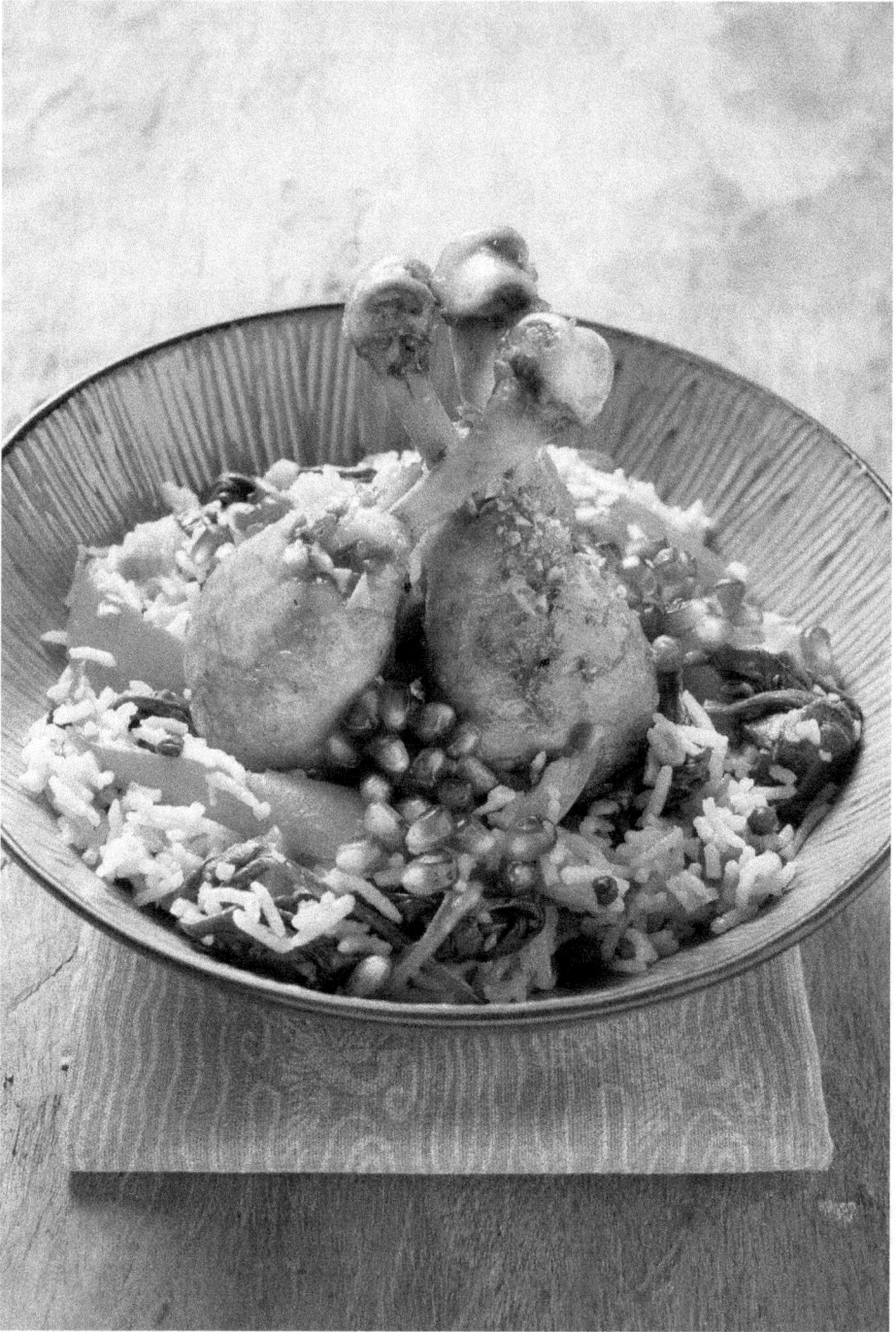

Chicken With Artichokes And Beans

Servings: 4

Cooking Time: 40 Minutes

Ingredients:

- 2 tablespoons olive oil
- 2 chicken breasts, skinless, boneless and halved
- Zest of 1 lemon, grated
- 3 garlic cloves, crushed
- Juice of 1 lemon
- Salt and black pepper to the taste
- 1 tablespoon thyme, chopped
- 6 ounces canned artichokes hearts, drained
- 1 cup canned fava beans, drained and rinsed
- 1 cup chicken stock
- A pinch of cayenne pepper
- Salt and black pepper to the taste

Directions:

1. Heat up a pan with the oil over medium-high heat, add chicken and brown for 5 minutes.
2. Add lemon juice, lemon zest, salt, pepper and the rest of the ingredients, bring to a simmer and cook over medium heat for 35 minutes.
3. Divide the mix between plates and serve right away.

Nutrition Info: calories 291, fat 14.9, fiber 10.5, carbs 23.8, protein 24.2

Chicken Pie

Servings: 6

Cooking Time: 50 Minutes

Ingredients:
- ¼ cup green peas, frozen
- 1 carrot, chopped
- 1 cup ground chicken
- 5 oz puff pastry
- 1 tablespoon butter, melted
- ¼ cup cream
- 1 teaspoon ground black pepper
- 1 oz Parmesan, grated

Directions:
1. Roll up the puff pastry and cut it on 2 parts.
2. Place one puff pastry part in the non-sticky springform pan and flatten.
3. Then mix up together green peas, chopped carrot, ground chicken, and ground black pepper.
4. Place the chicken mixture in the puff pastry.
5. Pour cream over mixture and sprinkle with Parmesan.
6. Cover the mixture with second puff pastry half and secure the edges of it with the help of the fork.

7. Brush the surface of the pie with melted butter and bake it for 50 minutes at 365F.

Nutrition Info:Per Serving:calories 223, fat 14.3, fiber 1, carbs 13.2, protein 10.5

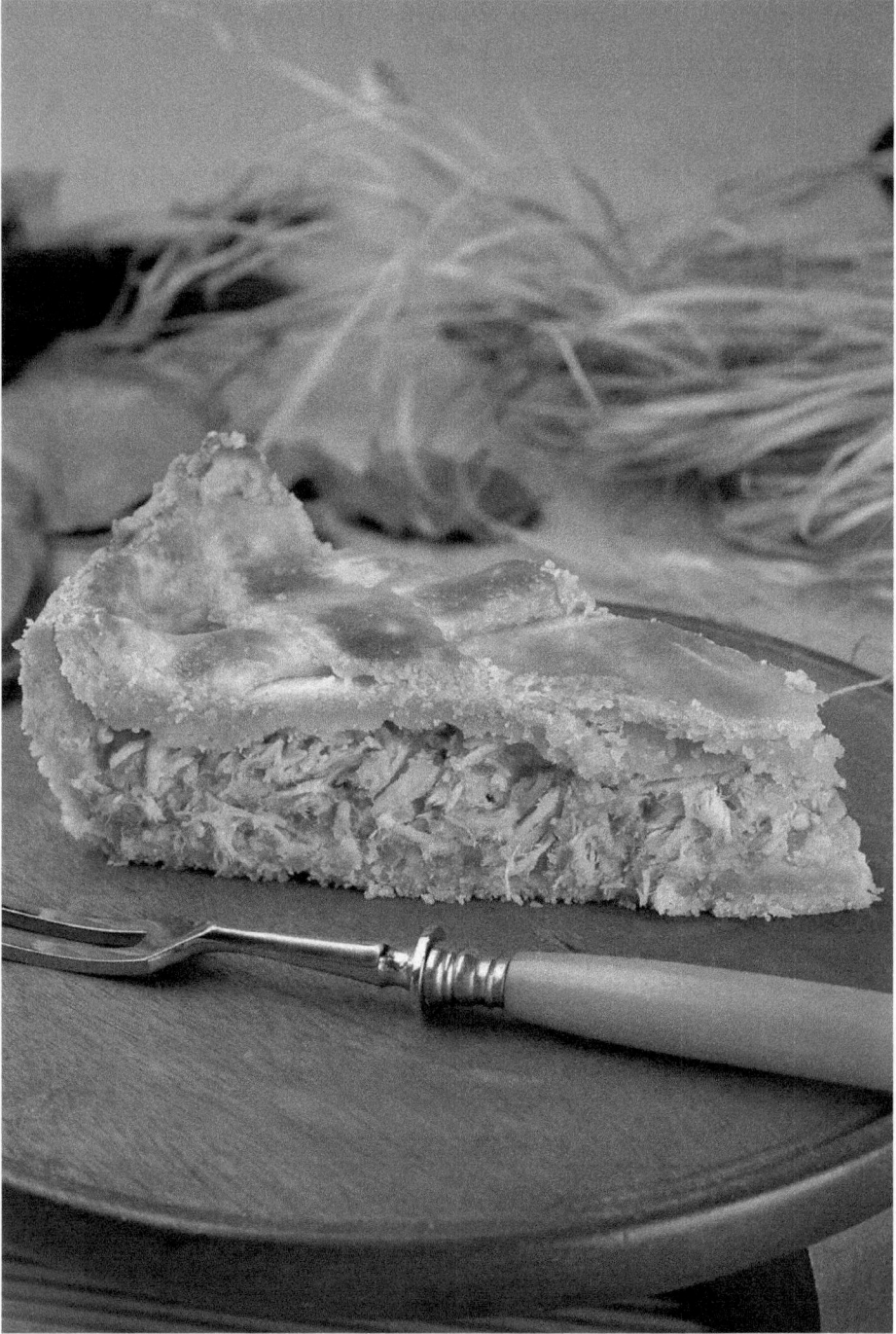

Chicken And Semolina Meatballs

Servings: 8

Cooking Time: 10 Minutes

Ingredients:

- 1/3 cup carrot, grated
- 1 onion, diced
- 2 cups ground chicken
- 1 tablespoon semolina
- 1 egg, beaten
- ½ teaspoon salt
- 1 teaspoon dried oregano
- 1 teaspoon dried cilantro
- 1 teaspoon chili flakes
- 1 tablespoon coconut oil

Directions:

1. In the mixing bowl combine together grated carrot, diced onion, ground chicken, semolina, egg, salt, dried oregano, cilantro, and chili flakes.

2. With the help of scooper make the meatballs.

3. Heat up the coconut oil in the skillet.

4. When it starts to shimmer, put meatballs in it.

5. Cook the meatballs for 5 minutes from each side over the medium-low heat.

Nutrition Info:Per Serving:calories 102, fat 4.9, fiber 0.5, carbs 2.9, protein 11.2

Lemon Chicken Mix

Servings: 2
Cooking Time: 10 Minutes

Ingredients:
- 8 oz chicken breast, skinless, boneless
- 1 teaspoon Cajun seasoning
- 1 teaspoon balsamic vinegar
- 1 teaspoon olive oil
- 1 teaspoon lemon juice

Directions:
1. Cut the chicken breast on the halves and sprinkle with Cajun seasoning.
2. Then sprinkle the poultry with olive oil and lemon juice.
3. Then sprinkle the chicken breast with the balsamic vinegar.
4. Preheat the grill to 385F.
5. Grill the chicken breast halves for 5 minutes from each side.
6. Slice Cajun chicken and place in the serving plate.

Nutrition Info:Per Serving:calories 150, fat 5.2, fiber 0, carbs 0.1, protein 24.1

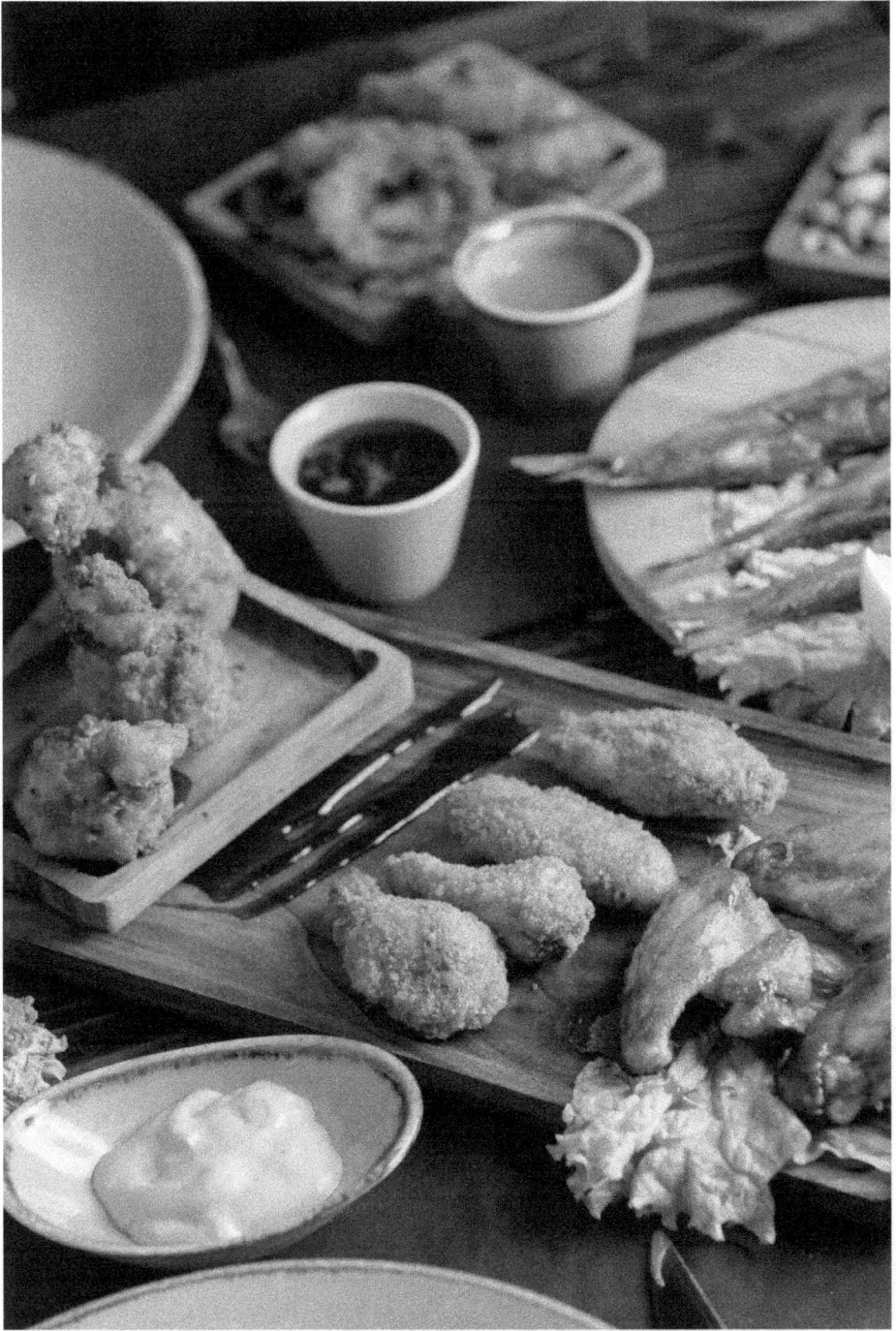

Turkey And Chickpeas

Servings: 4

Cooking Time: 5 Hours

Ingredients:

- 2 tablespoons avocado oil
- 1 big turkey breast, skinless, boneless and roughly cubed
- Salt and black pepper to the taste
- 1 red onion, chopped
- 15 ounces canned chickpeas, drained and rinsed
- 15 ounces canned tomatoes, chopped
- 1 cup kalamata olives, pitted and halved
- 2 tablespoons lime juice
- 1 teaspoon oregano, dried

Directions:

1. Heat up a pan with the oil over medium-high heat, add the meat and the onion, brown for 5 minutes and transfer to a slow cooker.

2. Add the rest of the ingredients, put the lid on and cook on High for 5 hours.

3. Divide between plates and serve right away!

Nutrition Info: calories 352, fat 14.4, fiber 11.8, carbs 25.1, protein 26.4

Cardamom Chicken And Apricot Sauce

Servings: 4

Cooking Time: 7 Hours

Ingredients:

- Juice of ½ lemon
- Zest of ½ lemon, grated
- 2 teaspoons cardamom, ground
- Salt and black pepper to the taste
- 2 chicken breasts, skinless, boneless and halved
- 2 tablespoons olive oil
- 2 spring onions, chopped
- 2 tablespoons tomato paste
- 2 garlic cloves, minced
- 1 cup apricot juice
- ½ cup chicken stock
- ¼ cup cilantro, chopped

Directions:

1. In your slow cooker, combine the chicken with the lemon juice, lemon zest and the other ingredients except the cilantro, toss, put the lid on and cook on Low for 7 hours.
2. Divide the mix between plates, sprinkle the cilantro on top and serve.

Nutrition Info: calories 323, fat 12, fiber 11, carbs 23.8, protein 16.4

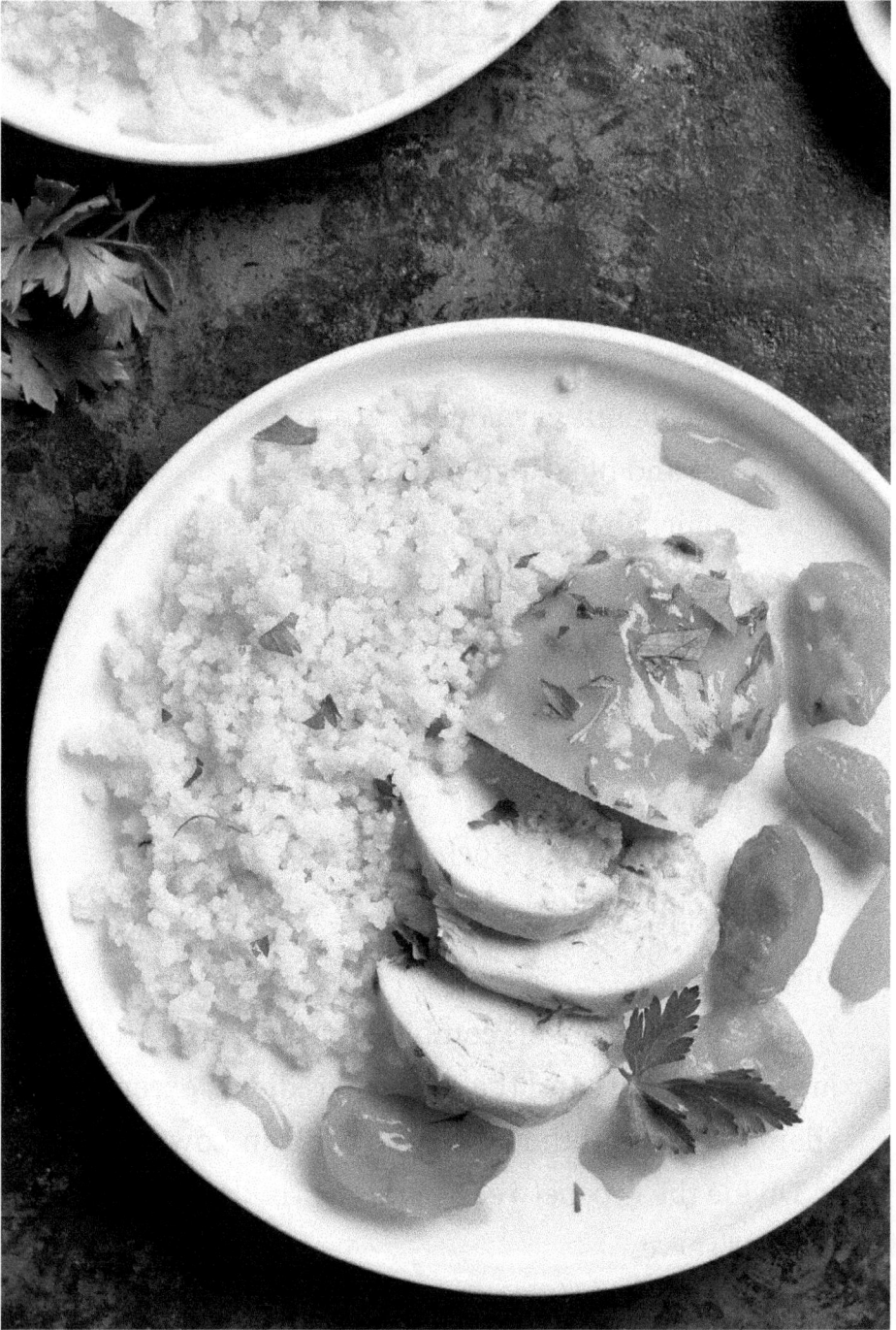

Chicken And Artichokes

Servings: 4

Cooking Time: 20 Minutes

Ingredients:

- 2 pounds chicken breast, skinless, boneless and sliced
- A pinch of salt and black pepper
- 4 tablespoons olive oil
- 8 ounces canned roasted artichoke hearts, drained
- 6 ounces sun-dried tomatoes, chopped
- 3 tablespoons capers, drained
- 2 tablespoons lemon juice

Directions:

1. Heat up a pan with half of the oil over medium-high heat, add the artichokes and the other ingredients except the chicken, stir and sauté for 10 minutes.
2. Transfer the mix to a bowl, heat up the pan again with the rest of the oil over medium-high heat, add the meat and cook for 4 minutes on each side.
3. Return the veggie mix to the pan, toss, cook everything for 2-3 minutes more, divide between plates and serve.

Nutrition Info: calories 552, fat 28, fiber 6, carbs 33, protein 43

Buttery Chicken Spread

Servings: 6

Cooking Time: 20 Minutes

Ingredients:

- 8 oz chicken liver
- 3 tablespoon butter
- 1 white onion, chopped
- 1 bay leaf
- 1 teaspoon salt
- ½ teaspoon ground black pepper
- ½ cup of water

Directions:

1. Place the chicken liver in the saucepan.
2. Add onion, bay leaf, salt, ground black pepper, and water.
3. Mix up the mixture and close the lid.
4. Cook the liver mixture for 20 minutes over the medium heat.
5. Then transfer it in the blender and blend until smooth.
6. Add butter and mix up until it is melted.
7. Pour the pate mixture in the pate ramekin and refrigerate for 2 hours.

Nutrition Info:Per Serving:calories 122, fat 8.3, fiber 0.5, carbs 2.3, protein 9.5

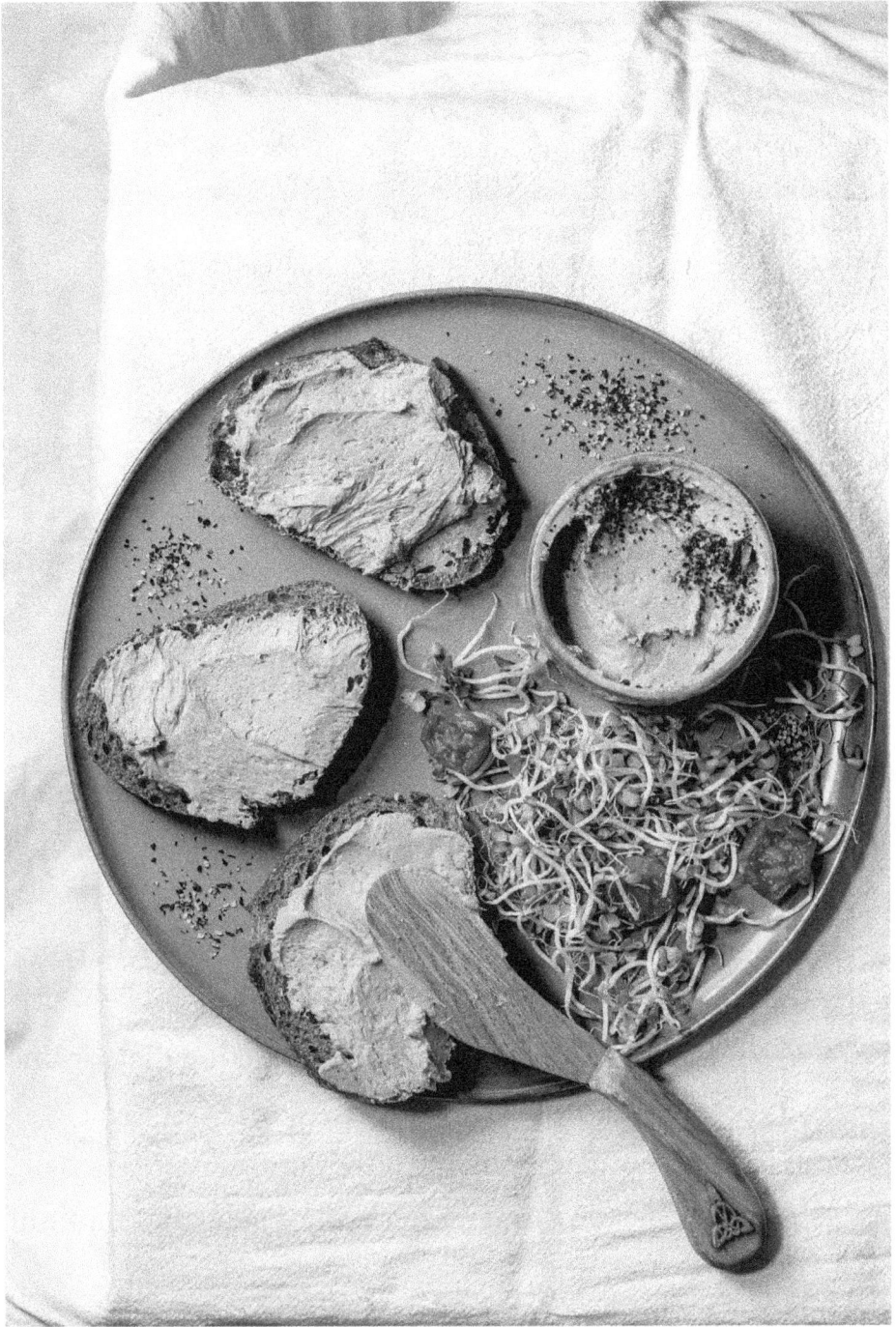

Chicken And Spinach Cakes

Servings: 4

Cooking Time: 15 Minutes

Ingredients:

- 8 oz ground chicken
- 1 cup fresh spinach, blended
- 1 teaspoon minced onion
- ½ teaspoon salt
- 1 red bell pepper, grinded
- 1 egg, beaten
- 1 teaspoon ground black pepper
- 4 tablespoons Panko breadcrumbs

Directions:

1. In the mixing bowl mix up together ground chicken, blended spinach, minced garlic, salt, grinded bell pepper, egg, and ground black pepper.

2. When the chicken mixture is smooth, make 4 burgers from it and coat them in Panko breadcrumbs.

3. Place the burgers in the non-sticky baking dish or line the baking tray with baking paper.

4. Bake the burgers for 15 minutes at 365F.

5. Flip the chicken burgers on another side after 7 minutes of cooking.

Nutrition Info:Per Serving:calories 171, fat 5.7, fiber 1.7, carbs 10.5, protein 19.4

Cream Cheese Chicken

Servings: 2

Cooking Time: 20 Minutes

Ingredients:
- 1 onion, chopped
- 1 sweet red pepper, roasted, chopped
- 1 cup spinach, chopped
- ½ cup cream
- 1 teaspoon cream cheese
- 1 tablespoon olive oil
- ½ teaspoon ground black pepper
- 8 oz chicken breast, skinless, boneless, sliced

Directions:

1. Mix up together sliced chicken breast with ground black pepper and put in the saucepan.

2. Add olive oil and mix up.

3. Roast the chicken for 5 minutes over the medium-high heat. Stir it from time to time.

4. After this, add chopped sweet pepper, onion, and cream cheese.

5. Mix up well and bring to boil.

6. Add spinach and cream. Mix up well.

7. Close the lid and cook chicken Alfredo for 10 minutes more over the medium heat.

Nutrition Info:Per Serving:calories 279, fat 14, fiber 2.5, carbs 12.4, protein 26.4

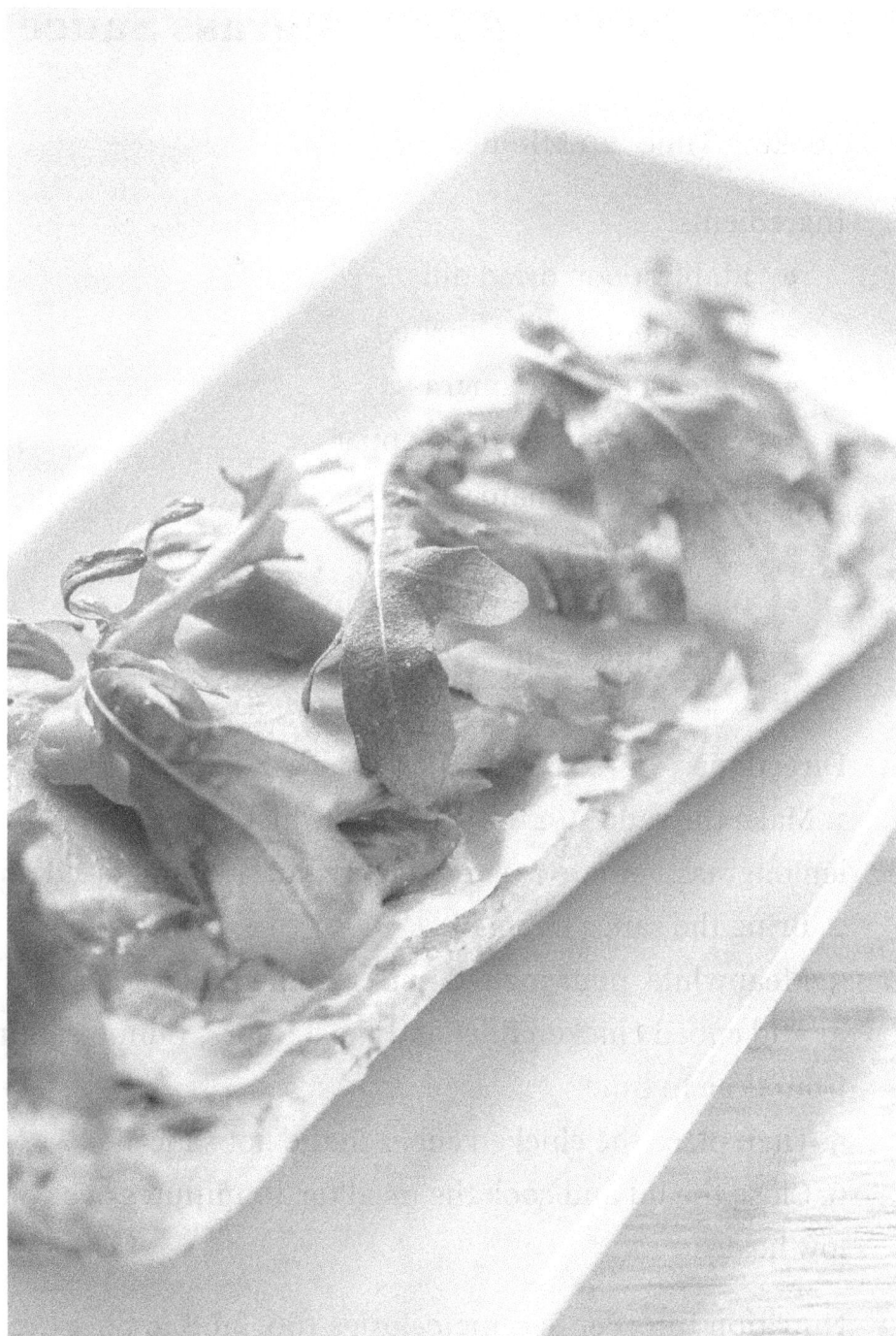

Chicken And Lemongrass Sauce

Servings: 4

Cooking Time: 20 Minutes

Ingredients:

- 1 tablespoon dried dill
- 1 teaspoon butter, melted
- ½ teaspoon lemongrass
- ½ teaspoon cayenne pepper
- 1 teaspoon tomato sauce
- 3 tablespoons sour cream
- 1 teaspoon salt
- 10 oz chicken fillet, cubed

Directions:

1. Make the sauce: in the saucepan whisk together lemongrass, tomato sauce, sour cream, salt, and dried dill.
2. Bring the sauce to boil.
3. Meanwhile, pour melted butter in the skillet.
4. Add cubed chicken fillet and roast it for 5 minutes. Stir it from time to time.
5. Then place the chicken cubes in the hot sauce.
6. Close the lid and cook the meal for 10 minutes over the low heat.

Nutrition Info:Per Serving:calories 166, fat 8.2, fiber 0.2, carbs 1.1, protein 21 3

Spiced Chicken Meatballs

Servings: 4

Cooking Time: 20 Minutes

Ingredients:
- 1 pound chicken meat, ground
- 1 tablespoon pine nuts, toasted and chopped
- 1 egg, whisked
- 2 teaspoons turmeric powder
- 2 garlic cloves, minced
- Salt and black pepper to the taste
- 1 and ¼ cups heavy cream
- 2 tablespoons olive oil
- ¼ cup parsley, chopped
- 1 tablespoon chives, chopped

Directions:

1. In a bowl, combine the chicken with the pine nuts and the rest of the ingredients except the oil and the cream, stir well and shape medium meatballs out of this mix.

2. Heat up a pan with the oil over medium-high heat, add the meatballs and cook them for 4 minutes on each side.

3. Add the cream, toss gently, cook everything over medium heat for 10 minutes more, divide between plates and serve.

Nutrition Info: calories 283, fat 9.2, fiber 12.8, carbs 24.4, protein 34.5

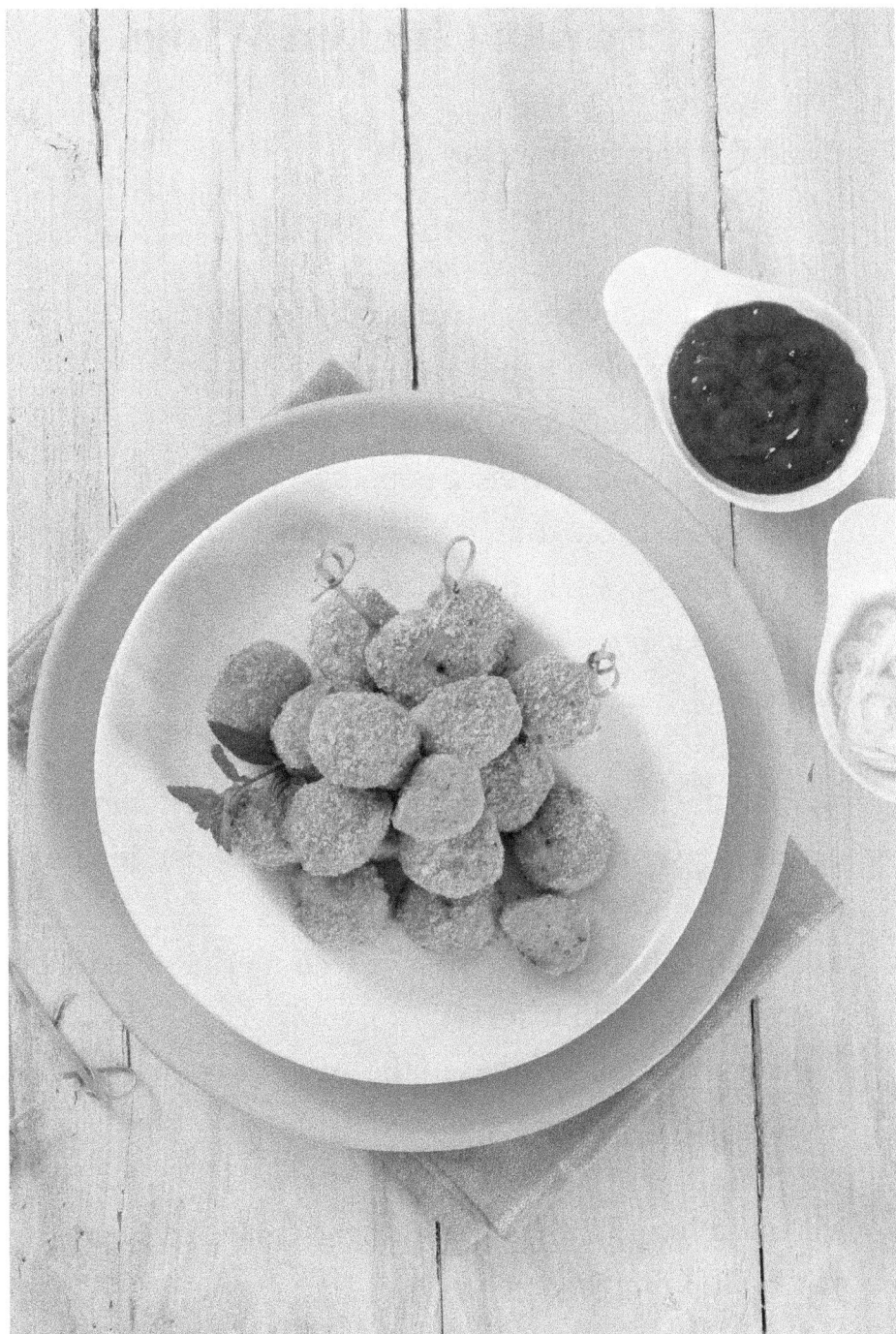

Paprika Chicken Wings

Servings: 4

Cooking Time: 8 Minutes

Ingredients:

- 4 chicken wings, boneless
- 1 tablespoon honey
- ½ teaspoon paprika
- ¼ teaspoon cayenne pepper
- ¾ teaspoon ground black pepper
- 1 tablespoon lemon juice
- ½ teaspoon sunflower oil

Directions:

1. Make the honey marinade: whisk together honey, paprika, cayenne pepper, ground black pepper, lemon juice, and sunflower oil.
2. Then brush the chicken wings with marinade carefully.
3. Preheat the grill to 385F.
4. Place the chicken wings in the grill and cook them for 4 minutes from each side.

Nutrition Info:Per Serving:calories 26, fat 0.8, fiber 0.3, carbs 5.1, protein 0.3

Chicken And Parsley Sauce

Servings: 4

Cooking Time: 25 Minutes

Ingredients:

- 1 cup ground chicken
- 2 oz Parmesan, grated
- 1 tablespoon olive oil
- 2 tablespoons fresh parsley, chopped
- 1 teaspoon chili pepper
- 1 teaspoon paprika
- ½ teaspoon dried oregano
- ¼ teaspoon garlic, minced
- ½ teaspoon dried thyme
- 1/3 cup crushed tomatoes

Directions:

1. Heat up olive oil in the skillet.

2. Add ground chicken and sprinkle it with chili pepper, paprika, dried oregano, dried thyme, and parsley. Mix up well.

3. Cook the chicken for 5 minutes and add crushed tomatoes. Mix up well.

4. Close the lid and simmer the chicken mixture for 10 minutes over the low heat.

5. Then add grated Parmesan and mix up.

6. Cook chicken bolognese for 5 minutes more over the medium heat.

Nutrition Info:Per Serving:calories 154, fat 9.3, fiber 1.1, carbs 3, protein 15.4

Sage Turkey Mix

Servings: 4

Cooking Time: 40 Minutes

Ingredients:

- 1 big turkey breast, skinless, boneless and roughly cubed
- Juice of 1 lemon
- 2 tablespoons avocado oil
- 1 red onion, chopped
- 2 tablespoons sage, chopped
- 1 garlic clove, minced
- 1 cup chicken stock

Directions:

1. Heat up a pan with the avocado oil over medium-high heat, add the turkey and brown for 3 minutes on each side.
2. Add the rest of the ingredients, bring to a simmer and cook over medium heat for 35 minutes.
3. Divide the mix between plates and serve with a side dish.

Nutrition Info: calories 382, fat 12.6, fiber 9.6, carbs 16.6, protein 33.2

Chipotle Turkey And Tomatoes

Servings: 4

Cooking Time: 1 Hour

Ingredients:

- 2 pounds cherry tomatoes, halved
- 3 tablespoons olive oil
- 1 red onion, roughly chopped
- 1 big turkey breast, skinless, boneless and sliced
- 3 garlic cloves, chopped
- 3 red chili peppers, chopped
- 4 tablespoons chipotle paste
- Zest of ½ lemon, grated
- Juice of 1 lemon
- Salt and black pepper to the taste
- A handful coriander, chopped

Directions:

1. Heat up a pan with the oil over medium-high heat, add the turkey slices, cook for 4 minutes on each side and transfer to a roasting pan.
2. Heat up the pan again over medium-high heat, add the onion, garlic and chili peppers and sauté for 2 minutes.
3. Add chipotle paste, sauté for 3 minutes more and pour over the turkey slices.

4. Toss the turkey slices with the chipotle mix, also add the rest of the ingredients except the coriander, introduce in the oven and bake at 400 degrees F for 45 minutes.
5. Divide everything between plates, sprinkle the coriander on top and serve.

Nutrition Info: calories 264, fat 13.2, fiber 8.7, carbs 23.9, protein 33.2

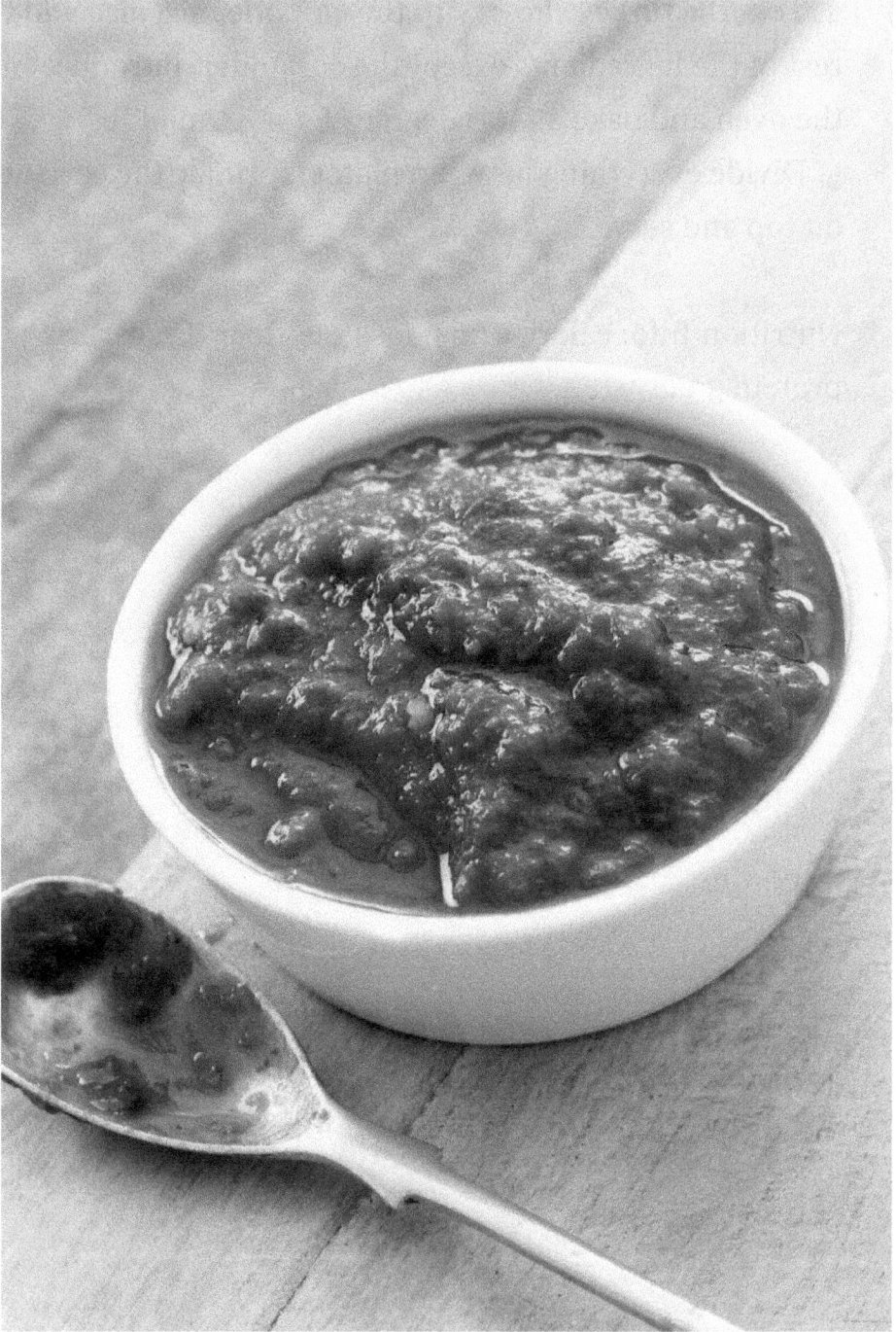

Curry Chicken, Artichokes And Olives

Servings: 6

Cooking Time: 7 Hours

Ingredients:

- 2 pounds chicken breasts, boneless, skinless and cubed
- 12 ounces canned artichoke hearts, drained
- 1 cup chicken stock
- 1 red onion, chopped
- 1 tablespoon white wine vinegar
- 1 cup kalamata olives, pitted and chopped
- 1 tablespoon curry powder
- 2 teaspoons basil, dried
- Salt and black pepper to the taste
- ¼ cup rosemary, chopped

Directions:

1. In your slow cooker, combine the chicken with the artichokes, olives and the rest of the ingredients, put the lid on and cook on Low for 7 hours.

2. Divide the mix between plates and serve hot.

Nutrition Info: calories 275, fat 11.9, fiber 7.6, carbs 19.7, protein 18.7

Roasted Chicken

Servings: ¼ Chicken

Cooking Time: 1 Hour 15 Minutes

Ingredients:

- 1 (5-lb.) whole chicken
- 1 TB. extra-virgin olive oil
- 2 TB. minced garlic
- 1 tsp. salt
- 1 tsp. paprika
- 1 tsp. black pepper
- 1 tsp. ground coriander
- 1 tsp. seven spices
- 1/2 tsp. ground cinnamon
- 1/2 large lemon, cut in 1/2
- 1/2 large yellow onion, cut in 1/2
- 2 sprigs fresh rosemary
- 2 sprigs fresh thyme
- 2 sprigs fresh sage
- 2 large carrots, cut into 1-in. pieces
- 6 small red potatoes, washed and cut in 1/2
- 4 cloves garlic

Directions:

1. Preheat the oven to 450°F. Wash chicken and pat dry with paper towels. Place chicken in a roasting pan, and drizzle and then rub chicken with extra-virgin olive oil.

2. In a small bowl, combine garlic, salt, paprika, black pepper, coriander, seven spices, and cinnamon. Sprinkle and then rub entire chicken with spice mixture to coat.

3. Place 1/4 lemon, 1/4 yellow onion, 1 sprig rosemary, 1 sprig thyme, and 1 sprig sage in chicken cavity.

4. Place remaining rosemary, thyme, sage, lemon, and onion around chicken in the roasting pan. Add carrots, red potatoes, and garlic cloves to the roasting pan.

5. Roast for 15 minutes. Reduce temperature to 375°F, and roast for 1 more hour, basting chicken every 20 minutes.

6. Let chicken rest for 15 minutes before serving.

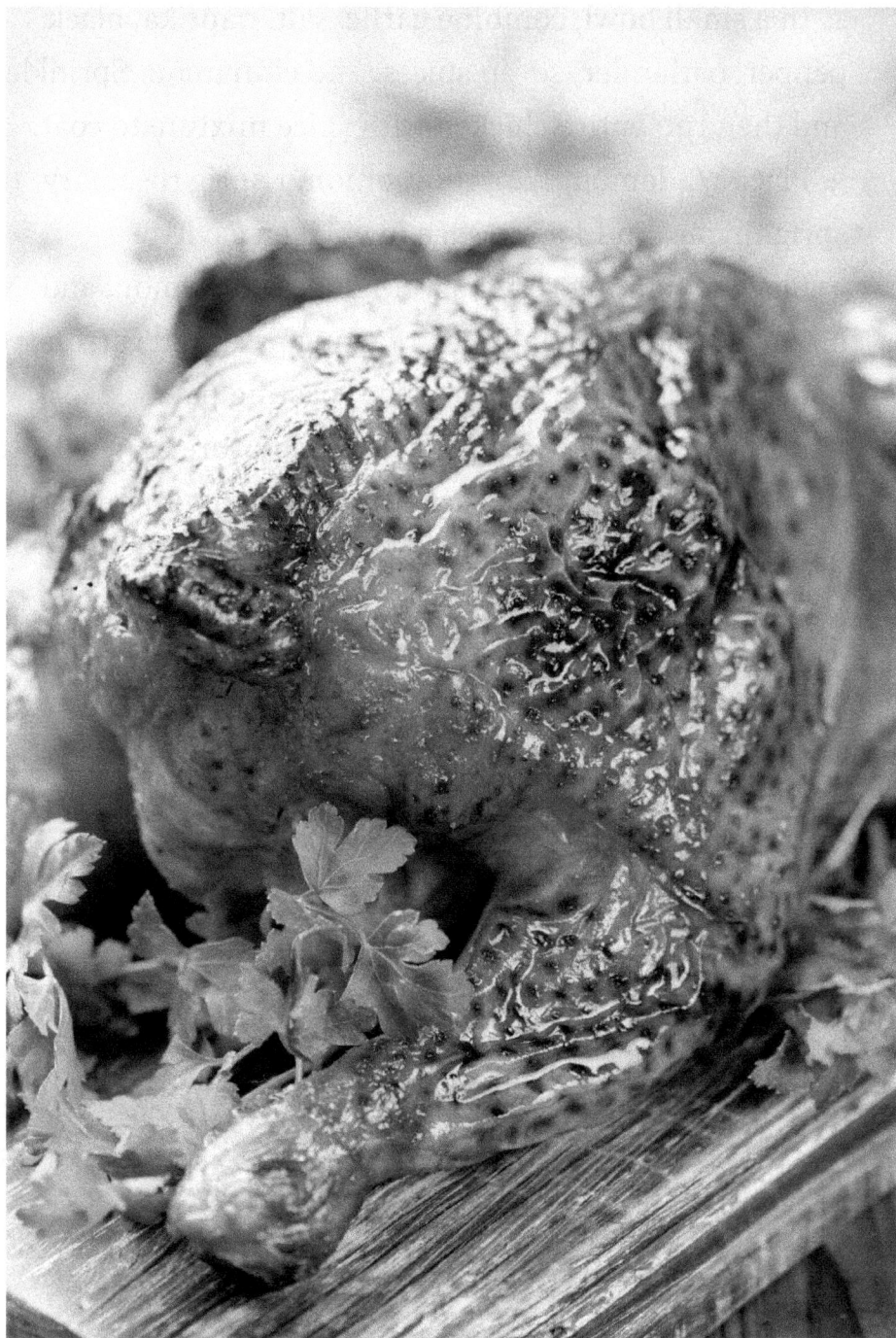

Curry Chicken Mix

Servings: 2

Cooking Time: 25 Minutes

Ingredients:

- 2 flatbread
- 7 oz chicken fillet
- 1 tablespoon yogurt
- 1 teaspoon minced garlic
- 1 teaspoon fresh parsley
- ½ teaspoon salt
- ½ teaspoon paprika
- ¼ teaspoon curry powder
- 1 tablespoon tomato sauce

Directions:

1. Make the marinade: mix up together yogurt, minced garlic, salt, paprika, and curry powder.
2. Chop the chicken fillet on the medium cubes and put them in the marinade.
3. Mix up the chicken well and leave to marinate for at least 15 minutes.
4. Then put the marinated chicken in the baking tray in one layer and bake it for 25 minutes at 350F. Flip the chicken on another side after 10 minutes of cooking.

5. Then put the cooked chicken on the flatbread and sprinkle with tomato sauce and parsley.

Nutrition Info:Per Serving:calories 290, fat 10.1, fiber 2.4, carbs 15.9, protein 32.5

Creamy Chicken

Servings: 4

Cooking Time: 35 Minutes

Ingredients:

- 1-pound chicken breast, skinless, boneless
- 3 oz Mozzarella, sliced
- 1 tomato, sliced
- 1 teaspoon Italian seasoning
- ½ teaspoon salt
- 1 tablespoon sour cream
- 1 teaspoon olive oil

Directions:

1. Make the cuts in the chicken breast in the shape of Hasselback.

2. Sprinkle the chicken with Italian seasoning, salt, and sour cream.

3. Massage the chicken breast gently.

4. Fill every chicken breast cut with sliced Mozzarella and sliced tomato.

5. Arrange the chicken breast in the baking dish and sprinkle it with olive oil.

6. Bake the chicken Hasselback for 35 minutes at 355F.

Nutrition Info:Per Serving:calories 212, fat 8.8, fiber 0.2, carbs 1.6, protein 30.3

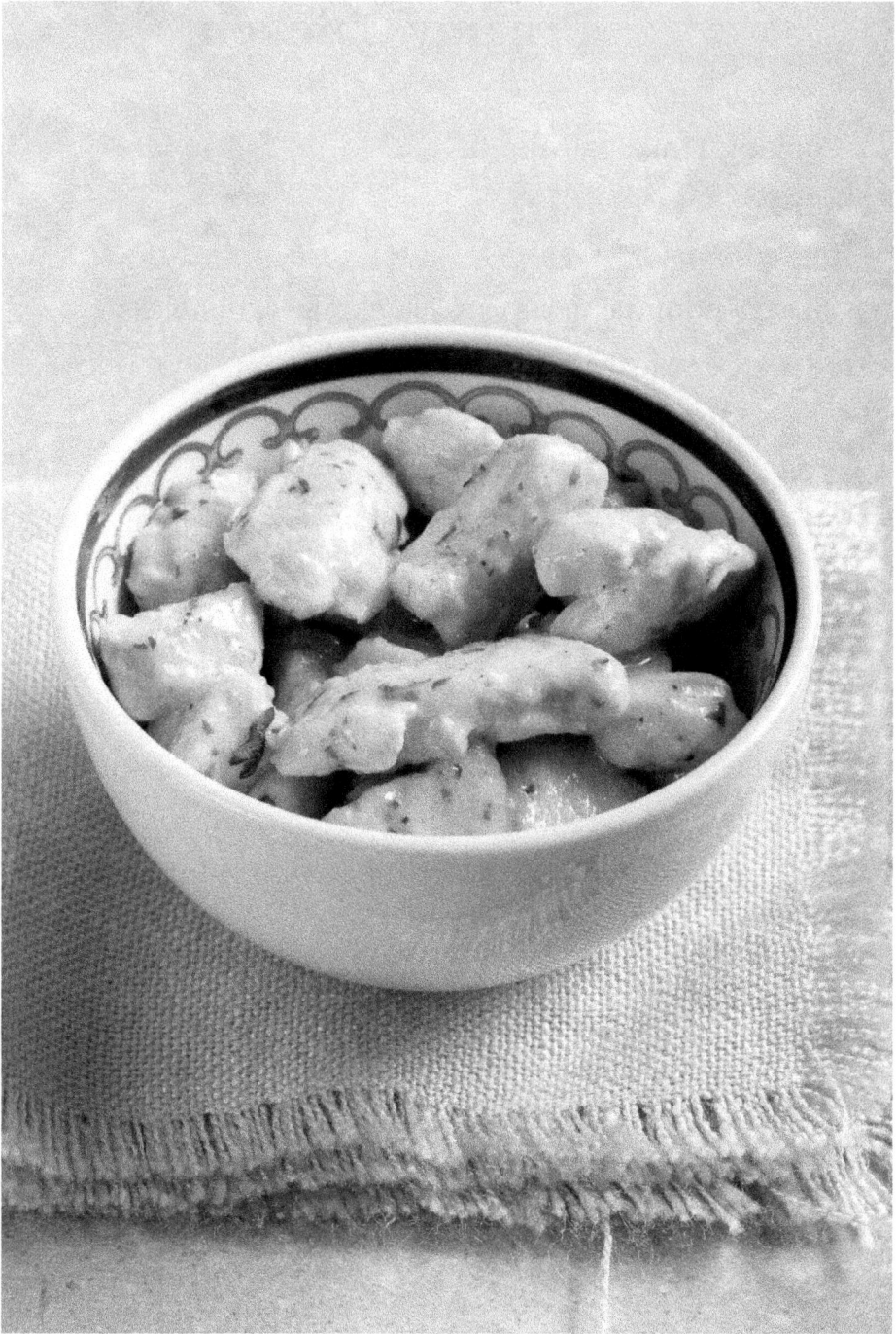

Chicken And Celery Quinoa Mix

Servings: 4

Cooking Time: 50 Minutes

Ingredients:

- 4 chicken things, skinless and boneless
- 1 tablespoon olive oil
- Salt and black pepper to the taste
- 2 celery stalks, chopped
- 2 spring onions, chopped
- 2 cups chicken stock
- ½ cup cilantro, chopped
- ½ cup quinoa
- 1 teaspoon lime zest, grated

Directions:

1. Heat up a pot with the oil over medium-high heat, add the chicken and brown for 4 minutes on each side.
2. Add the onion and the celery, stir and sauté everything for 5 minutes more.
3. Add the rest of the ingredients, toss, bring to a simmer and cook over medium-low heat for 35 minutes.
4. Divide everything between plates and serve.

Nutrition Info: calories 241, fat 12.6, fiber 9.5, carbs 15.6, protein 34.1

Turmeric Chicken And Eggplant Mix

Servings: 4

Cooking Time: 30 Minutes

Ingredients:

- 2 cups eggplant, cubed
- Salt and black pepper to the taste
- 2 tablespoons olive oil
- 1 cup yellow onion, chopped
- 2 tablespoons garlic, minced
- 2 tablespoons hot paprika
- 1 teaspoon turmeric powder
- 1 and ½ tablespoons oregano, chopped
- 1 cup chicken stock
- 1 pound chicken breast, skinless, boneless and cubed
- 1 cup half and half
- 1 tablespoon lemon juice

Directions:

1. Heat up a pan with the oil over medium-high heat, add the chicken and brown for 4 minutes on each side.

2. Add the eggplant, onion and garlic and sauté for 5 minutes more.

3. Add the rest of the ingredients, bring to a simmer and cook over medium

heat for 16 minutes.

4. Divide the mix between plates and serve.

Nutrition Info: calories 392, fat 11.6, fiber 8.3, carbs 21.1, protein 24.2

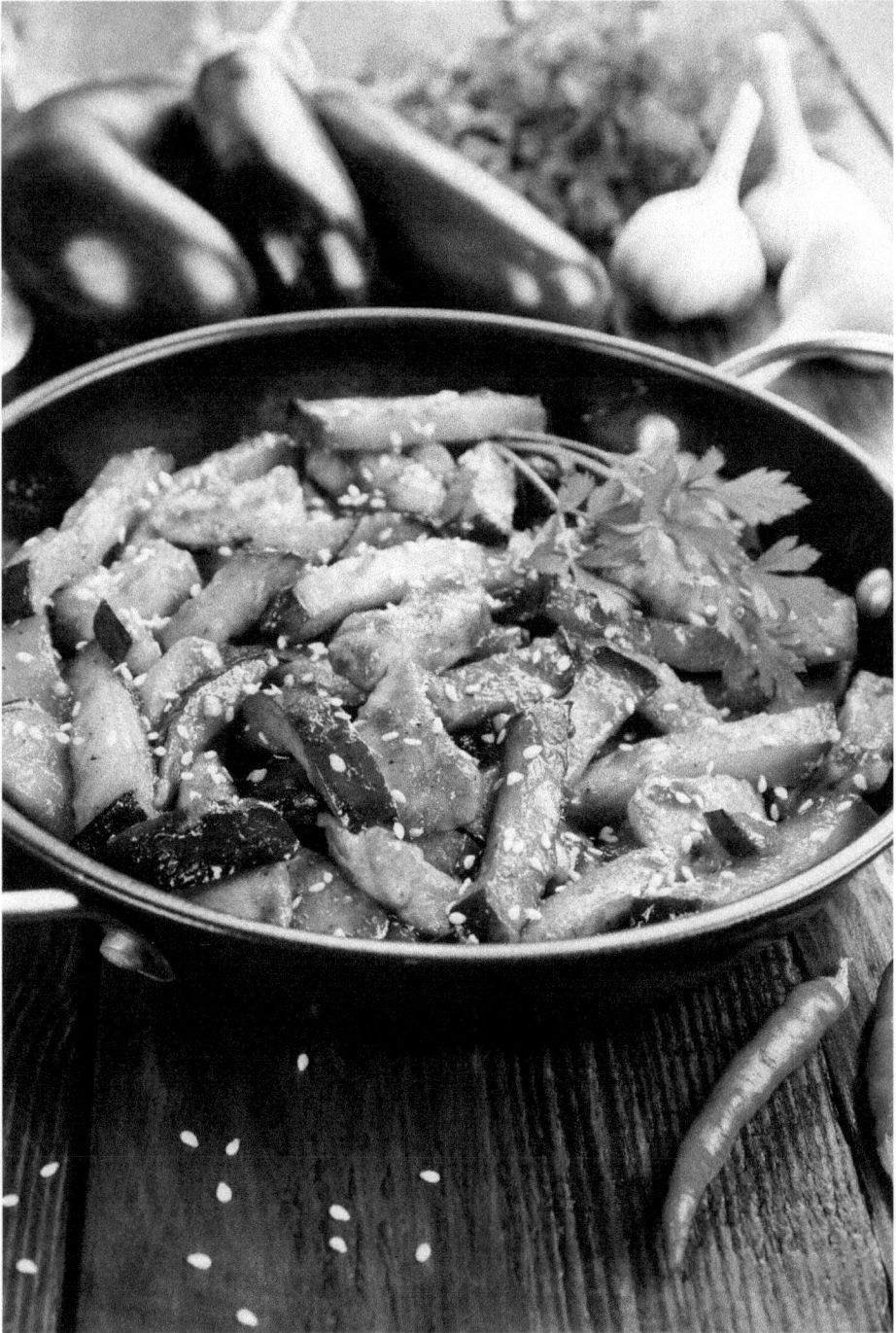

Honey Chicken

Servings: 5

Cooking Time: 25 Minutes

Ingredients:

- 5 chicken drumsticks
- 2 oz currant
- ½ teaspoon liquid honey
- 1 teaspoon butter
- 1 teaspoon lime juice
- ½ teaspoon salt
- ¼ cup of water
- ½ teaspoon chili pepper

Directions:

1. Mix up together chicken drumsticks with chili pepper and salt.

2. Put butter in the skillet and heat it up.

3. Add chicken drumsticks and cook them for 15 minutes or until they are cooked.

4. Meanwhile, mash currant and mix it up with lime juice, liquid honey, and water.

5. Pour the currant mixture over the drumstick and close the lid.

6. Cook the meal for 5 minutes over the medium heat.

Nutrition Info:Per Serving:calories 93, fat 3.4, fiber 0.5, carbs 2.2, protein 12.8

Chicken And Nutmeg Butter Sauce

Servings: 4

Cooking Time: 30 Minutes

Ingredients:
- 4 chicken thighs, skinless, boneless
- 1 teaspoon ground black pepper
- ½ teaspoon salt
- 1 teaspoon paprika
- ¼ cup Cheddar cheese, shredded
- 1 tablespoon cream cheese
- ½ teaspoon garlic powder
- 1 teaspoon fresh dill, chopped
- 1 tablespoon butter
- 1 teaspoon olive oil
- ½ teaspoon ground nutmeg

Directions:

1. Grease the baking dish with butter.

2. Then heat up olive oil in the skillet.

3. Meanwhile, rub the chicken thighs with ground nutmeg, garlic powder, paprika, and salt. Add ground black pepper.

4. Roast the chicken thighs in the hot oil over the high heat for 2 minutes from each side.

5. Then transfer the chicken thighs in the prepared baking dish.

6. Mix up together Cheddar cheese, cream cheese, and dill.

7. Top every chicken thigh with cheese mixture and bake for 25 minutes at 365F.

Nutrition Info:Per Serving:calories 79, fat 7.5, fiber 0.4, carbs 1.2, protein 2.4

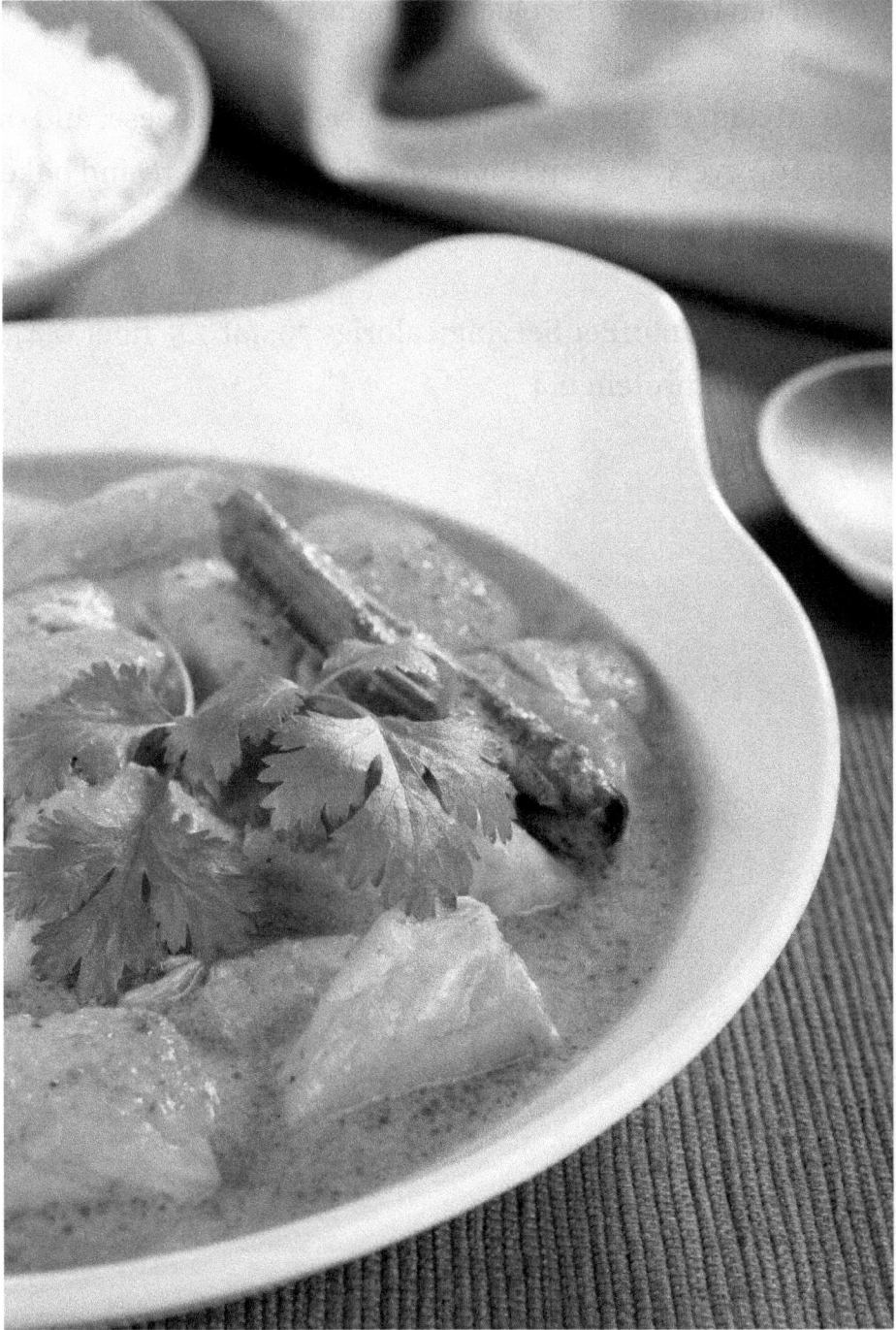

Cheddar Chicken Mix

Servings: 4

Cooking Time: 20 Minutes

Ingredients:

- 4 chicken fillets (4 oz each fillet)
- 1 cup cherry tomatoes
- 1 tablespoon olive oil
- 1 tablespoon fresh basil, chopped
- ½ teaspoon salt
- ½ teaspoon ground black pepper
- 1 teaspoon balsamic vinegar
- 1 teaspoon garlic clove, diced
- 1 oz Cheddar cheese, shredded

Directions:

1. Pour olive oil in the skillet and heat it up.

2. Sprinkle the chicken fillets with salt and ground black pepper and put in the hot oil.

3. Roast the chicken for 3 minutes from each side over the medium heat.

4. Then cut the cherry tomatoes on the halves and add in the olive oil.

5. Sprinkle the vegetables with balsamic vinegar, garlic, and basil.

6. Mix up the ingredients well.

7. Sprinkle the chicken with Cheddar cheese and close the lid.

8. Cook the chicken caprese for 10 minutes over the medium heat.

Nutrition Info:Per Serving:calories 299, fat 17, fiber 1.6, carbs 17.3, protein 21.3

Chicken And Veggie Saute

Servings: 2

Cooking Time: 25 Minutes

Ingredients:

- 4 oz chicken fillet
- 4 tomatoes, peeled
- 1 bell pepper, chopped
- 1 teaspoon olive oil
- 1 cup of water
- 1 teaspoon salt
- 1 chili pepper, chopped
- ½ teaspoon saffron

Directions:

1. Pour water in the pan and bring it to boil.

2. Meanwhile, chop the chicken fillet.

3. Add the chicken fillet in the boiling water and cook it for 10 minutes or until the chicken is tender.

4. After this, put the chopped bell pepper and chili pepper in the skillet.

5. Add olive oil and roast the vegetables for 3 minutes.

6. Add chopped tomatoes and mix up well.

7. Cook the vegetables for 2 minutes more.

8. Then add salt and a ¾ cup of water from chicken.

9. Add chopped chicken fillet and mix up.

10. Cook the saute for 10 minutes over the medium heat.

Nutrition Info:Per Serving:calories 192, fat 7.2, fiber 3.8, carbs 14.4, protein 19.2

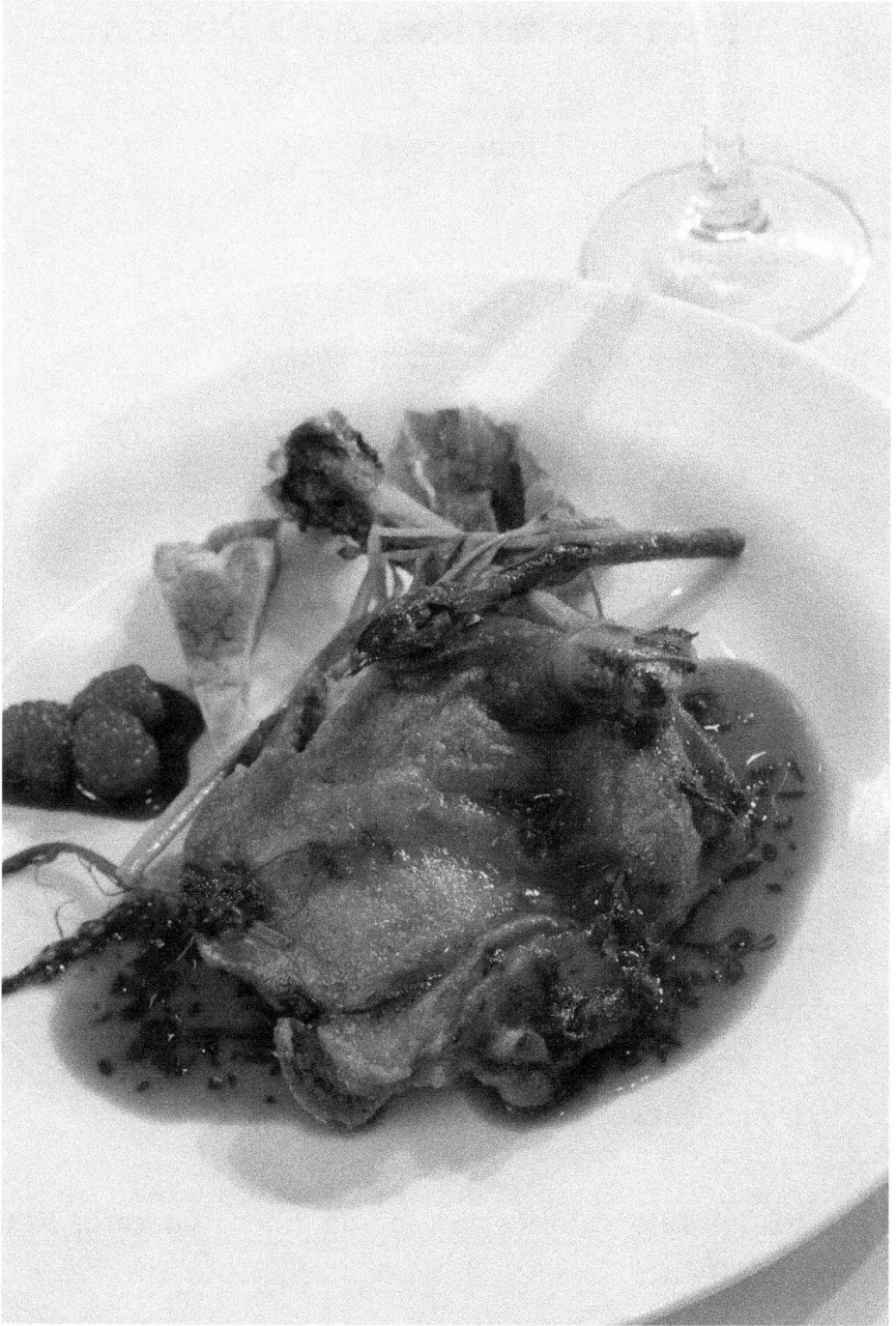

Thyme Chicken And Potatoes

Servings: 4

Cooking Time: 50 Minutes

Ingredients:

- 1 tablespoon olive oil
- 4 garlic cloves, minced
- A pinch of salt and black pepper
- 2 teaspoons thyme, dried
- 12 small red potatoes, halved
- 2 pounds chicken breast, skinless, boneless and cubed
- 1 cup red onion, sliced
- ¾ cup chicken stock
- 2 tablespoons basil, chopped

Directions:

1. In a baking dish greased with the oil, add the potatoes, chicken and the rest of the ingredients, toss a bit, introduce in the oven and bake at 400 degrees F for 50 minutes.
2. Divide between plates and serve.

Nutrition Info: calories 281, fat 9.2, fiber 10.9, carbs 21.6, protein 13.6

Creamy Chicken And Mushrooms

Servings: 4

Cooking Time: 30 Minutes

Ingredients:

- 1 red onion, chopped
- 1 tablespoon olive oil
- 2 garlic cloves, minced
- 2 carrots chopped
- Salt and black pepper to the taste
- 1 tablespoon thyme, chopped
- 1 and ½ cups chicken stock
- ½ pound Bella mushrooms, sliced
- 1 cup heavy cream
- 2 chicken breasts, skinless, boneless and cubed
- 2 tablespoons chives, chopped
- 1 tablespoon parsley, chopped

Directions:

1. Heat up a Dutch oven with the oil over medium-high heat, add the onion and the garlic and sauté for 5 minutes.
2. Add the chicken and the mushrooms, and sauté for 10 minutes more.

3. Add the rest of the ingredients except the chives and the parsley, bring to a simmer and cook over medium heat for 15 minutes.

4. Add the chives and parsley, divide the mix between plates and serve.

Nutrition Info: calories 275, fat 11.9, fiber 10.6, carbs 26.7, protein 23.7

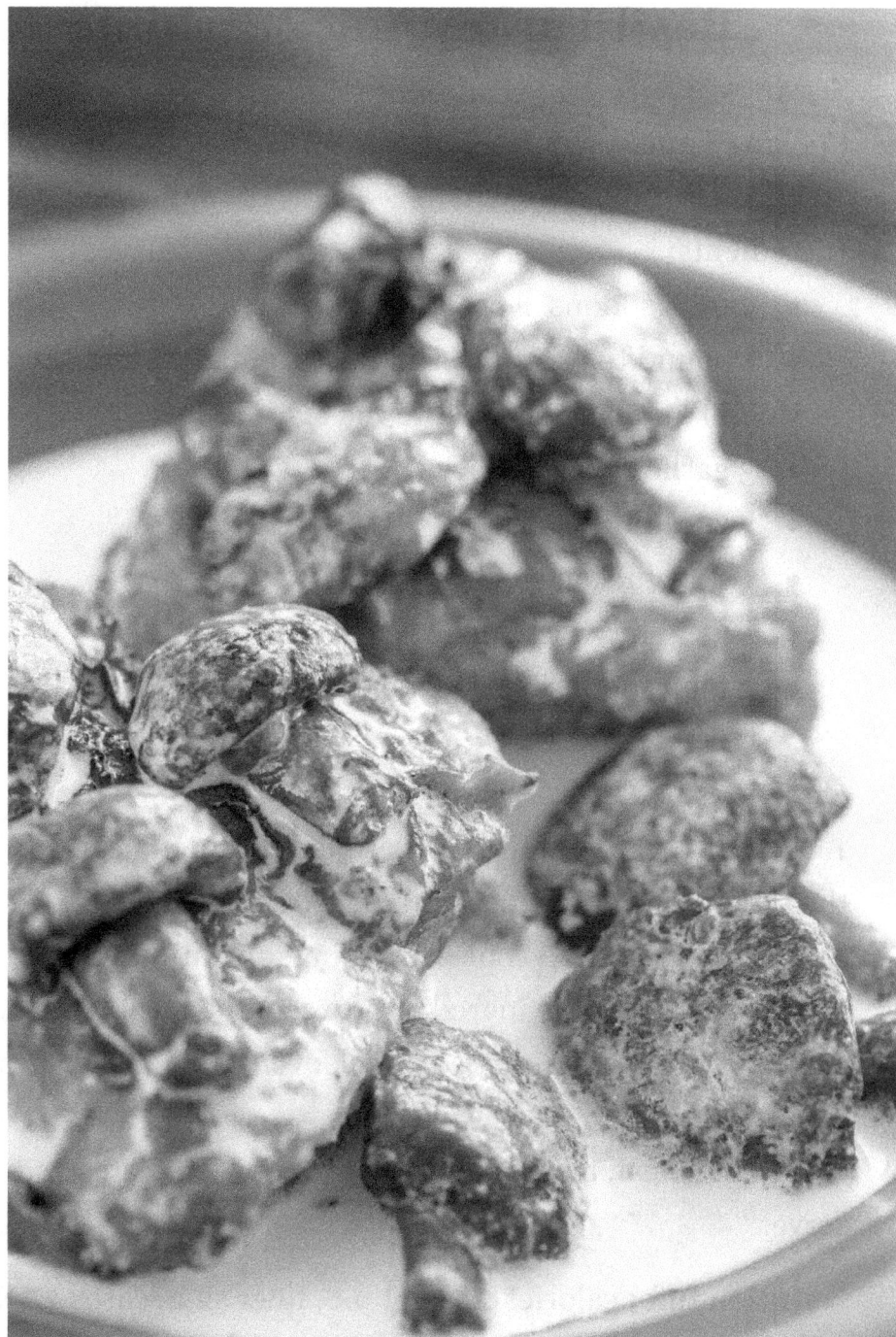

Basil Turkey And Zucchinis

Servings: 4

Cooking Time: 1 Hour

Ingredients:

- 2 tablespoons avocado oil
- 1 pound turkey breast, skinless, boneless and sliced
- Salt and black pepper to the taste
- 3 garlic cloves, minced
- 2 zucchinis, sliced
- 1 cup chicken stock
- ¼ cup heavy cream
- 2 tablespoons basil, chopped

Directions:

1. Heat up a pot with the oil over medium-high heat, add the turkey and brown for 5 minutes on each side.

2. Add the garlic and cook everything for 1 minute.

3. Add the rest of the ingredients except the basil, toss gently, bring to a simmer and cook over medium-low heat for 50 minutes.

4. Add the basil, toss, divide the mix between plates and serve.

Nutrition Info: calories 262, fat 9.8, fiber 12.2, carbs 25.8, protein 14.6

Herbed Almond Turkey

Servings: 4

Cooking Time: 40 Minutes

Ingredients:

- 1 big turkey breast, skinless, boneless and cubed
- 1 tablespoon olive oil
- ½ cup chicken stock
- 1 tablespoon basil, chopped
- 1 tablespoon rosemary, chopped
- 1 tablespoon oregano, chopped
- 1 tablespoon parsley, chopped
- 3 garlic cloves, minced
- ½ cup almonds, toasted and chopped
- 3 cups tomatoes, chopped

Directions:

1. Heat up a pan with the oil over medium-high heat, add the turkey and the garlic and brown for 5 minutes.

2. Add the stock and the rest of the ingredients, bring to a simmer over medium heat and cook for 35 minutes.

3. Divide the mix between plates and serve.

Nutrition Info: calories 297, fat 11.2, fiber 9.2, carbs 19.4, protein 23.6

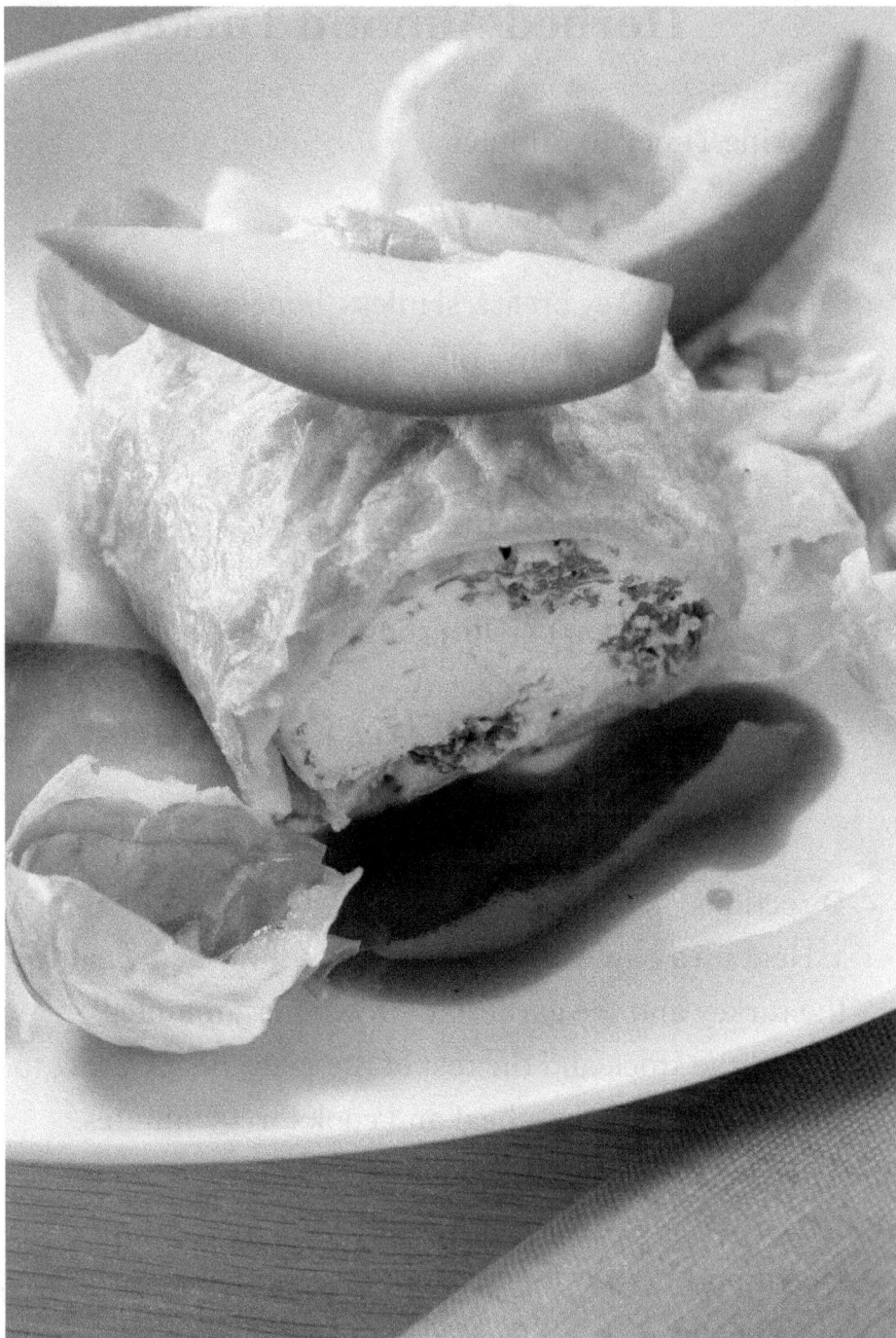

Lime Chicken Thighs And Pomegranate Sauce

Servings: 2

Cooking Time: 10 Minutes

Ingredients:

- 1 tablespoon pomegranate molasses
- 8 oz chicken thighs (4 oz each chicken thigh)
- ½ teaspoon paprika
- 1 teaspoon cornstarch
- ½ teaspoon chili flakes
- ½ teaspoon ground black pepper
- 1 teaspoon olive oil
- ½ teaspoon lime juice

Directions:

1. In the shallow bowl mix up together ground black pepper, chili flakes, paprika, and cornstarch.
2. Rub the chicken thighs with spice mixture.
3. Heat up olive oil in the skillet.
4. Add chicken thighs and roast them for 4 minutes from each side over the medium heat.
5. When the chicken thighs are light brown, sprinkle them with pomegranate molasses and roast for 1 minute from each side.

Nutrition Info:Per Serving:calories 353, fat 21, fiber 0.4, carbs 9.3, protein 30.2 358.

Mediterranean Meatloaf

Servings: 1/8 Loaf

Cooking Time: 45 Minutes

Ingredients:

- 2 lb. ground chicken
- 1/3 cup plain breadcrumbs
- 11/2 tsp. salt
- 1 tsp. garlic powder
- 1 tsp. ground black pepper
- 1 tsp. paprika
- 1/2 tsp. dried oregano
- 1/2 tsp. dried thyme
- 2 TB. fresh basil, chopped
- 2 TB. fresh Italian parsley, chopped
- 1 large egg
- 1 large carrot, shredded
- 1 cup fresh or frozen green peas
- 1/2 cup sun-dried tomatoes, chopped
- 1 cup ketchup

Directions:

1. Preheat the oven to 400°F. Lightly coat all sides of a 9×5-inch loaf pan with olive oil spray.

2. In a large bowl, combine chicken, breadcrumbs, salt, garlic powder, black pepper, paprika, oregano, thyme, basil, Italian parsley, egg, carrot, green peas, and sun-dried tomatoes.

3. Transfer chicken mixture to the prepared pan, and even out top. Cover the pan with a piece of aluminum foil, and bake for 40 minutes.

4. After 40 minutes have passed, pour ketchup over top of loaf and spread out evenly. Bake for 5 more minutes.

5. Remove meatloaf from the oven, and let rest for 10 minutes before slicing and serving warm.

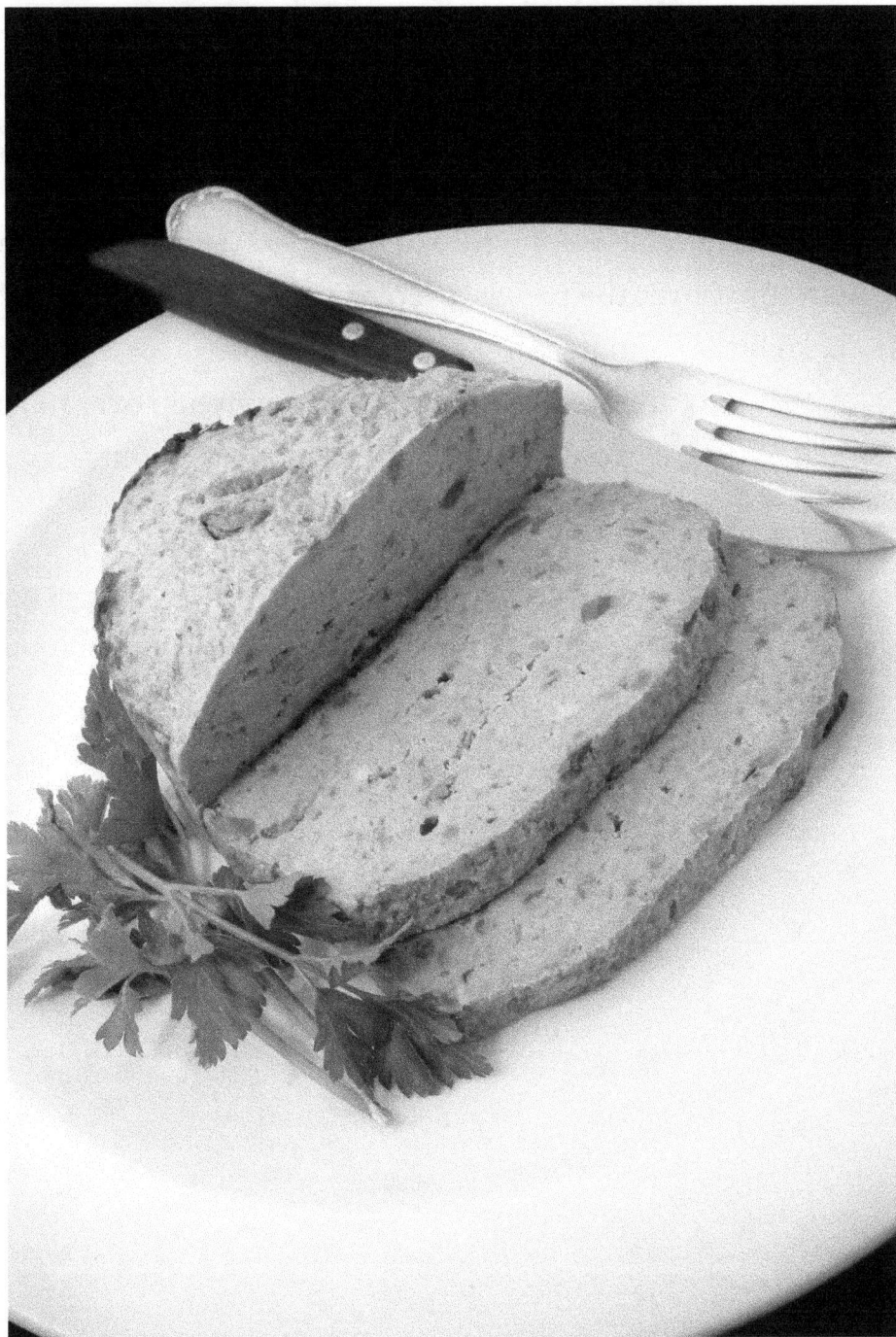

Lemon Chicken

Servings: 4

Cooking Time: 20 Minutes

Ingredients:

- 1-pound chicken breast, skinless, boneless
- 3 tablespoons lemon juice
- 1 tablespoon olive oil
- 1 teaspoon ground black pepper

Directions:

1. Cut the chicken breast on 4 pieces.

2. Sprinkle every chicken piece with olive oil, lemon juice, and ground black pepper.

3. Then place them in the skillet.

4. Roast the chicken for 20 minutes over the medium heat.

5. Flip the chicken pieces every 5 minutes.

Nutrition Info:Per Serving:calories 163, fat 6.5, fiber 0.2, carbs 0.6, protein 24.2

Chicken And Mushroom Mix

Servings: 2

Cooking Time: 20 Minutes

Ingredients:

- 9 oz chicken fillet, cubed
- 1/3 cup cream
- ¼ cup mushrooms, chopped
- 1 teaspoon butter
- ½ onion, diced
- ½ teaspoon ground black pepper
- ½ teaspoon salt
- 1 teaspoon hot pepper
- 1 teaspoon sunflower oil

Directions:

1. Sprinkle the chicken cubes with hot pepper and mix up.
2. Pour sunflower oil in the skillet and roast chicken cubes for 5 minutes over the medium heat. Stir them from time to time.
3. Toss butter in the separated skillet and melt it.
4. Add mushrooms and sprinkle them with salt and ground black pepper. 5. Add onion.
6. Cook the vegetables for 10 minutes over the low heat. Stir them with the help of spatula every 3 minutes.

7. Then add cream and bring to boil.

8. Add roasted chicken cubes and mix up well.

9. Close the lid and simmer the meal for 5 minutes.

Nutrition Info:Per Serving:calories 213, fat 10.7, fiber 0.5, carbs 3, protein 25.2

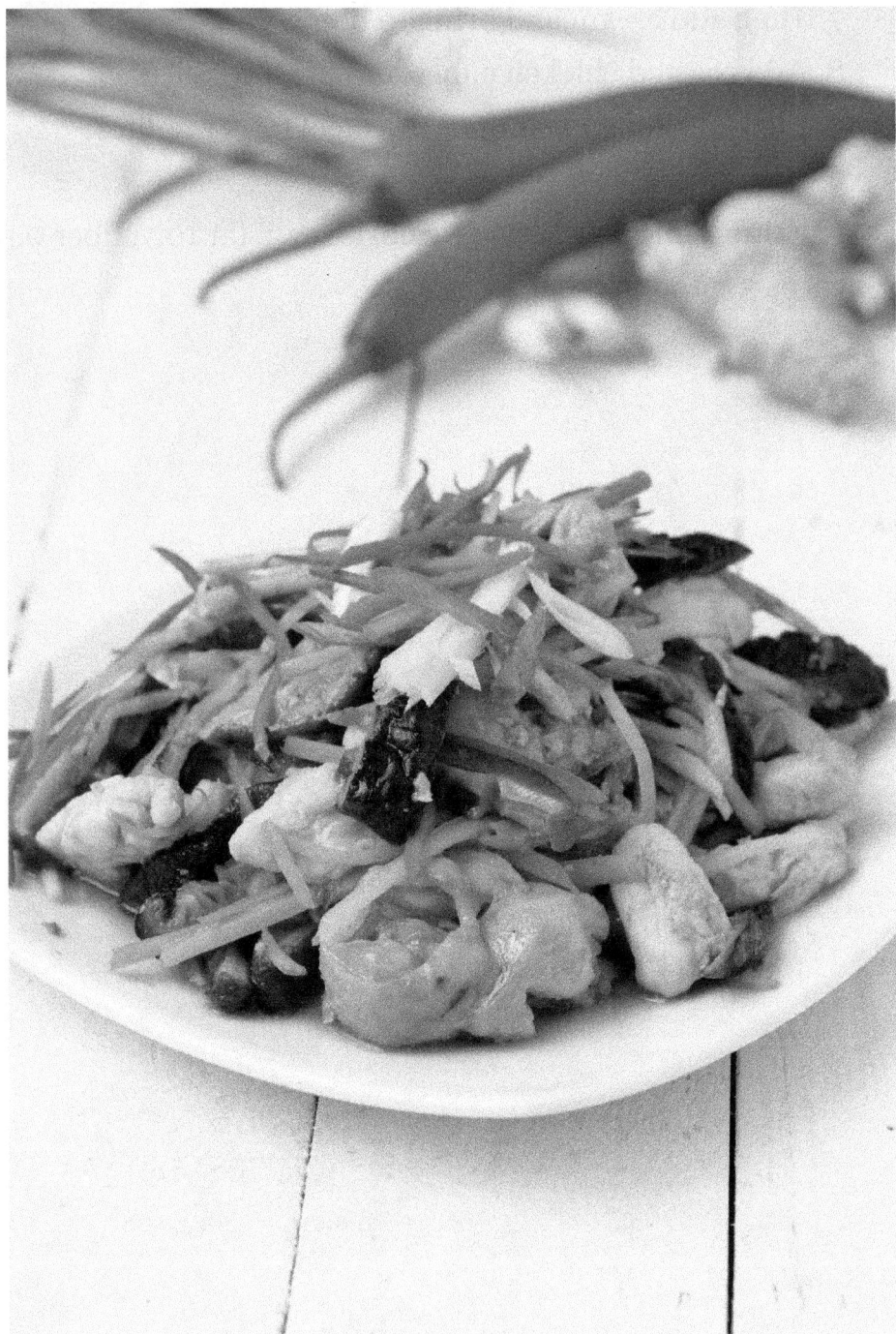

Chicken And Ginger Cucumbers Mix

Servings: 4

Cooking Time: 20 Minutes

Ingredients:

- 4 chicken breasts, boneless, skinless and cubed
- 2 cucumbers, cubed
- Salt and black pepper to the taste
- 1 tablespoon ginger, grated
- 1 tablespoon garlic, minced
- 2 tablespoons balsamic vinegar
- 3 tablespoons olive oil
- ¼ teaspoon chili paste
- ½ cup chicken stock
- ½ tablespoon lime juice
- 1 tablespoon chives, chopped

Directions:

1. Heat up a pan with the oil over medium-high heat, add the chicken and brown for 3 minutes on each side.

2. Add the cucumbers, salt, pepper and the rest of the ingredients except the chives, bring to a simmer and cook over medium heat for 15 minutes.

3. Divide the mix between plates and serve with the chives sprinkled on top.

Nutrition Info: calories 288, fat 9.5, fiber 12.1, carbs 25.6, protein 28.6

Dill Chicken Stew

Servings: 2

Cooking Time: 25 Minutes

Ingredients:

- 1 ½ cup water
- 6 oz chicken fillet
- 1 chili pepper, chopped
- 1 onion, diced
- 1 teaspoon butter
- ½ teaspoon salt
- ½ teaspoon paprika
- 1 tablespoon fresh dill, chopped

Directions:

1. Pour water in the saucepan.

2. Add chicken fillet and salt. Boil it for 15 minutes over the medium heat.

3. Then remove the chicken fillet from water and shred it with the help of the fork.

4. Return it back in the hot water.

5. Melt butter in the skillet and add diced onion. Roast it until light brown and transfer in the shredded chicken.

6. Add paprika, dill, chili pepper, and mix up.

7. Close the lid and simmer Posole for 5 minutes.

8. Ladle it in the serving bowls.

Nutrition Info:Per Serving:calories 207, fat 8.4, fiber 1.7, carbs 6.5, protein 25.7

Notes

www.ingramcontent.com/pod-product-compliance
Lightning Source LLC
Chambersburg PA
CBHW050759030426
42336CB00012B/1874